Manual on
COSMETIC GYNECOLOGY

AF647687

Manual on

COSMETIC GYNECOLOGY

Series Editors

Nandita Palshetkar
MD FCPS FICOG FRCOG (UK)
Professor Emeritus
Department of Obstetrics and Gynecology
DY Patil School of Medicine
Navi Mumbai, Maharashtra, India
Founder and Medical Director of the
Famous Bloom IVF Group

Hrishikesh D Pai
MD FRCOG (UK-HON) FCPS FICOG MSc (USA)
Trustee, FIGO, Asia Oceania (2023–25)
Professor, DY Patil University
Navi Mumbai, Maharashtra, India
Immediate Past President FOGSI (2022–23)
Founder and Medical Director
Bloom IVF Group, Mumbai

Niranjan Chavan
MD FICOG FCPS DGO DFP MICOG DICOG Diploma in Endoscopy (USA)
Professor and Unit Chief
Department of Obstetrics and Gynecology
Lokmanya Tilak Medical College and General Hospital
Mumbai, Maharashtra, India

Editors

Sejal Ajmera
MBBS MD DNB DHA FCPS DGO DFP
Professor, Aesthetic and Functional Gyne
DY Patil University
Consultant Obstetrician and Gynecologist
Surya Hospitals, Sujay Hospital and Criticare
Mumbai, Maharashtra, India

Neharika Malhotra MD (Gold Medalist)
DRM (Germany) DMIS FICMCH FMAS FICOG ICOG
Fellowship in Reproductive Medicine DGC
Consultant
Department of Obstetrics and Gynecology
Ujala Cygnus Rainbow Hospital
Agra, Uttar Pradesh, India

Apurba Kumar Dutta MBBS MS (Gold Medalist)
Consultant Cosmetic and Laparoscopic Gynecologist
Shree Durga Clinic and Fertility Centre
Dhanbad, Jharkhand, India
Chairperson, Sexual Health and STI Committee FOGSI

Co-Editors

Navneet Magon, Neeraj Jadhav, Suyesha Khanijao, Chandini Kharat, Zeel Shah, Snighda Kumar

JAYPEE BROTHERS MEDICAL PUBLISHERS
The Health Sciences Publisher
New Delhi | London

Message from Series Editors

Dear AICOG 2025 delegates,

It is a matter of great pride that the landmark AICOG 2025 is being held in the city of Mumbai, Maharashtra, India. The Organizing Committee and the hosts Mumbai Obstetric and Gynaecological Society have left no stone unturned in their quest to make this a historic event by aiming to have a scientific program of the highest caliber, punctuated by fantastic keynotes and orations, graced by the best international faculty in the field of Obstetrics, Gynecology and its subspecialities along with a cultural treat every evening to cater to the audience which hails from far-flung corners of India and the globe.

On this occasion, the academic stalwarts and senior FOGSIans have burned the midnight oil at both ends to contribute and create a set of AICOG 2025 Workshop Manuals that aim to amalgamate the most recent scientific advancements and evidence-based best practices in a nutshell for the delegates to take home and implement in their practices when they have returned from this magnificent event.

We acknowledge the efforts of all the editors, co-editors, authors, co-authors, co-contributors and junior authors who have sometimes worked at short notice to submit excellent chapters and articles included in the final publication. We also wish to take this opportunity to thank Shri Jitendar P Vij (Group Chairman) and Mr Ankit Vij (Managing Director) of M/s Jaypee Brothers Medical Publishers (P) Ltd, New Delhi, India, in publishing the book and their associates, particularly Ms Chetna Malhotra (Senior Director—Professional Publishing, Marketing, and Business Development), Ms Kritika Dua (Senior Commissiong Editor), and Mr Priyansh Saxena (Development Editor), who have been prompt, efficient, and most helpful.

We hope that the delegates and the attendees will enjoy reading this publication and the scientific data included therein will help to shape your knowledge, attitudes and practices and ultimately benefit the women of our country, whom we all serve.

Nandita Palshetkar
Organizing Chairperson, AICOG Mumbai, 2025

Hrishikesh D Pai
Chairperson, Scientific Committee, AICOG Mumbai, 2025

Niranjan Chavan
Organizing Secretary, AICOG Mumbai, 2025

Jaypee Brothers Medical Publishers (P) Ltd

Headquarters
EMCA House
23/23-B, Ansari Road, Daryaganj
New Delhi 110 002, India
Landline: +91-11-23272143, +91-11-23272703
+91-11-23282021, +91-11-23245672
E-mail: jaypee@jaypeebrothers.com

Corporate Office
4838/24, Ansari Road, Daryaganj
New Delhi 110 002, India
Phone: +91-11-43574357
Fax: +91-11-43574314
E-mail: jaypee@jaypeebrothers.com

Overseas Office
J.P. Medical Ltd
83 Victoria Street, London
SW1H 0HW (UK)
Phone: +44 20 3170 8910
E-mail: info@jpmedpub.com

EU GPSR Authorised Representative
Logos Europe, 9 rue Nicolas Poussin
17000, La Rochelle, France
Phone: +33 (0) 6 67 93 73 78
E-mail: contact@logoseurope.eu

Website: www.jaypeebrothers.com
Website: www.jaypeedigital.com

Inquiries for bulk sales may be solicited at: jaypee@jaypeebrothers.com

Manual on Cosmetic Gynecology

First Edition: 2025
Reprint: 2026
ISBN: 978-93-6616-313-0
Printed in India

Contributors

AL Satyavati MD DGO
Director and Senior Consultant
Srujana Multispeciality Hospital and IVF Centre
Kakinada, Andhra Pradesh, India

Bela Shah Jain
MBBS MS (Gold Medalist) DNB FMAS
Consultant Obstetrician & Gynecologist and Infertility Specialist
Laparoscopic Surgeon and Cosmetic Gynecologist
Asian Institute of Infertility Management
Indore, Madhya Pradesh, India

Deepali Gupta
MBBS MD (Obs & Gyne) FICS
Director
Ashirwad Multi Speciality Hospital
Varanasi, Uttar Pradesh, India

Jaideep Malhotra MD FICOG FICS FIUMB FICMCH FMAS FRCPI FRCOG FICRM
Managing Director
ART Rainbow IVF Infertility
Agra, Uttar Pradesh, India

Jay Mehta MBBS DNB
Scientific Director of Shree IVF and Endometriosis Clinic, Mumbai
Endometriosis Surgeon, Femmenest
New Delhi, India

Keshav Malhotra
Master of Clinical Embryology (MCE Australia) MBBS
Joint Treasurer- Delhi Chapter of ISAR (Indian Society of Assisted Reproduction)-(2015–2017)
National Committee Member– Quality Control and Accreditation Committee ISAR 2016 Onwards
Committee Member Quality Control and Accreditation ASPIRE 2016 Onwards
Member Managing Committee Indian Society of Assisted Reproduction 2018
Lab Director–Rainbow IVF, Agra (January 2015-Present)
Director– Global Rainbow Healthcare (January 2015–Present)
Director of Training Rainbow IVF (January 2015–Present)

Krupa Bhagat
MBBS MS
Aesthetic Vulvo-vaginal Surgeon
Dr Purvi Khatri Advanced Gynecology and Fertility Clinic
Surat, Gujrat, India

Maalavika Appasani
MS (Obs & Gyne)
Laparoscopic Surgeon
Aesthetic, Regenerative and Functional Gynecologist
Founder of Eternelle Aesthetics
Hyderabad, Telangana, India

Manish Mahajan
MBBS DGO DNB Fellowship in Cosmetic Gynecology (AAA)
Diploma in Cosmetic Gynecology (AAA) Fellowship in Stem Cells and Regenerative Medicine
Certified in Psychosexual Medicine (Mysore)
Director
Madalasaa Aesthetic Gynecology Center
Kalyan, Maharashtra, India

Manjula Anagani
MBBS MD (Obstetrics & Gynecology) FICOG
Padmashree Awardee
Clinical Director and HOD
Care and Arete Hospitals
Hyderabad, Telangana, India

Milind R Shah
MD DGO DFP FICOG FIAOG
President ISOPARB (2016–18)
2nd Vice President of FOGSI (2011)
Past Chairman-Rural Obstetrics Committee of FOGSI (2004–08)
Deputy Secretary General–InSARG (2022–2025)
Hon Secretary General
Federation of Asia Oceania Perinatal Societies (FAOPS)
President Elect, ISPAT
Professor and Head
Department of Obstetrics and Gynecologist
Gandhi Natha H Medical College
Peer Reviewer for Journal of Obstetrics and Gynecology of India

Muskan Mittal
MBBS Final Year PG Gynae
Senior Resident
The Touch Clinic (Advanced Gyne & IVF Centre)
Mohali, Punjab, India

Narendra Malhotra
MD FIAJAGO FICMU FICOG FICMCH FRCOG FICS FMAS AFIAPM FICRM
Managing Director
Global Rainbow Health Care and MNMH (P) Ltd and
Ujala Cygnus Rainbow Hospital
Agra, Uttar Pradesh, India

Naval Shah
MS DNB DRMS (Kiel, Germany)
Consultant Obstetrician and Gynecologist, Sonologist
Infertility Specialist and Cosmetic Gynecologist
Naval Nursing Home
Solapur, Maharashtra, India

Neharika Malhotra
MD (Gold Medalist) DRM (Germany) DMIS FICMCH FMAS FICOG ICOG Fellowship in Reproductive Medicine DGC
Consultant
Department of Obstetrics and Gynecology
Ujala Cygnus Rainbow Hospital
Agra, Uttar Pradesh, India

Parneet Kaur Sekhon
MBBS MS
Consultant
Kang Klinic
Mohali, Punjab, India

Parul Saoji
MBBS DNB MNAMS FMAS Diploma in Cosmetic and Gynecology
Cosmetic Gynecologist
Laparoscopic Surgeon
Infertility Specialist
Oracel Clinic
Nagpur, Maharashtra, India

Poonam
MBBS DGO MRCOG
Consultant
Apollo Cradle
Chirag Enclave
Delhi NCR, India

Prabhu Chandra Mishra
MSc–Molecular Medicine & Stemcell Technology
PG Diploma Chemoinformatics
PhD Researcher–Biotechnology (Regenerative Medicine)
President–International Association of Stemcell and Regenerative Medicine, New Delhi, India
StemMax Research and Therapeutics Pvt Ltd
New Delhi, India

Pragati Tandon BAMS
Resident
The Touch Clinic (Advanced Gynae & IVF Centre)
Mohali, Punjab, India

Preeti Jindal
MD DNB MRCOG (London) FICOG
Director – The Touch Clinic (Advanced Gyne and IVF Centre, Mohali)
High Risk Pregnancy
Recurrent Miscarriage Expert
IVF Treatment Specialist
Robotic Surgeon and Cosmetic Gynecologist
General Secretary–InSARG (Indian Aesthetic & Regenerative Gynecologists Society)
Past President–Mohali Obstetrics and Gynecology Society

Purvi Khatri
MBBS MD (Obstetrics and Gynecology)
Consultant
Dr Purvi Khatri Advanced Gynecology and Fertility Clinic
Surat, Gujrat, India

Rainee Agrawal MBBS MD FMAS
Consultant Gynecologist
Rainee's Clinic
Mumbai, Maharashtra, India

Ridhi Gulati MBBS MD (Gyne)
Consultant
The Touch Clinic (Advanced Gynae and IVF Centre)
Mohali, Punjab, India

Rupinder Kaur Ruprai
MBBS MD Assoc-RCOG FMAS DMIS D Repr Med M Cosmetic-Gyne, F RegenMed MBA
Health Bay Clinics
Al Wasl
Dubai, UAE

Savana Chongtham
MD
Urogynec and Feminine Aesthetic Surgeon
Founder and President
Savannah's She Matters Institute of Regenerative and Aesthetics
Founder and President
Asian Academy of Feminine Aesthetics
Founder KGlobal Academy of Feminine Aesthetics
Master Trainer and Thesis Guide
Post Doctoral Fellowship in Complete Feminine Aesthetics

Sebanti Goswami
MBBS MD (Obs & Gyne)
Consultant Gynecologist
Manipal Hospitals
Kolkata, West Bengal, India

Sejal Ajmera
MBBS MD DNB DHA FCPS DGO DFP
Professor
Aesthetic and Functional Gyne
DY Patil University
Consultant Obstetrician and Gynecologist
Surya Hospitals, Sujay Hospital and Criticare
Mumbai, Maharashtra, India

Sindura Gadde
MBBS MD
Consultant
Arete Hospitals
Hyderabad, Telangana, India

Sumitu Sahdev
MBBS PhD
Consultant
The Touch Clinic (Advanced Gyne & IVF Centre)
Mohali, Punjab, India

Surakshith Battina
MD
Managing Director Indigo Womens Center
Anna Nagar, Chennai, Tamil Nadu
Clinical Head Indian Endometriosis Foundation
Performed World's first "Laparoscopic Management of Uterine Rupture at 20 weeks"
TedX Speaker

Vidya Pancholia MBBS MS (Obs & Gyne) FICOG FICMCH Master Course on Cosmetic Vaginal Surgery and Laser Therapy (FDA Approved Er-YAG)
Senior Consultant
V-Care Laser Center
Indore, Madhya Pradesh, India

Preface

The manual on Cosmetic Gynecology for the workshop at AICOG 2025 has 20 elaborate chapters walking us through the entire armamentarium of history, surgeries, non-surgical procedures, regenerative techniques, and new updates.

The authors have painstakingly put together every chapter, starting from the basics to advanced understanding of every topic. We really appreciate the time, efforts, and a very special applause to all of them.

We deeply thank the entire FOGSI team for the unwavering faith shown in us. Special mention to Dr Hrishikesh D Pai, Dr Nandita Palshetkar, and Dr Niranjan Chavan. Thanks, Dr Rohan Palshetkar, for guiding this through completion.

Thank you, team Jaypee, without whom this would never have been possible. A huge shout out to Priyansh Saxena for the constant push, nudge, and a very professional way of seeing the manual through.

This is a relatively new subspeciality of ObGyn, which is now becoming popular and is really improving the intimate wellness and quality of life of our patients.

We wish the doctors happy reading and hope it ignites a thought that burns strong..

Hope you enjoy reading it as much as the joy it gave us writing it...

Series Editors: Nandita Palshetkar, Hrishikesh D Pai, Niranjan Chavan
Editors: Sejal Ajmera, Neharika Malhotra, Apurba Kumar Datta
Co-Editors: Navneet Magon, Neeraj Jadhav, Suyesha Khanijao, Chandini Kharat, Zeel Shah, Snighda Kumar

Contents

1

CHAPTER

History of Aesthetic and Functional Gynecology

Sejal Ajmera, Rainee Agrawal

INTRODUCTION

Cosmetic gynecology has evolved as an important field within women's health, blending aesthetic procedures with gynecological expertise. The roots of cosmetic gynecology, however, stretches back through centuries of cultural practices, medical advancements, and evolving societal norms related to female anatomy and beauty.

ADVENT AND EVOLUTION OF SURGICAL PROCEDURES

Surgical procedures for suturing vaginal lacerations postdelivery were first described by Trotula in 1050 AD in treatments for women.

In a study from India, female genital cosmetic surgery has increased by 30% from 2012 to 2016.[1]

Vaginoplasty

Vaginoplasty's roots trace to the mid-19th century, with J Marion Sims pioneering vesicovaginal fistula repair techniques.

In the late 1950s, Dr James Burt's controversial surgeries aimed to enhance women's sexual experiences, indirectly sparking interest in functional and aesthetic vaginal surgeries.

In the early 20th century, perineorrhaphy emerged, followed by posterior colporrhaphy in the mid-century, treating vaginal laxity and prolapse but not cosmetic concerns.

Aesthetic demands led to the advent of cosmetic vaginoplasty in the 1980s, popularized by gynecologists like Dr David Matlock (USA), who pioneered the use of lasers to perform precise incisions for vaginal tightening.[2]

Hymenoplasty

In the 1850s, a German physician, Dr Bernhard Sigmund Schultze, was one of the earliest to describe and document a hymen repair surgery particularly among women who feared social consequences due to the loss of virginity.[3]

The rise of the internet in the late 1990s and early 2000s facilitated the spread of information about hymenoplasty, making the procedure more accessible to women who were seeking it but did not know where to go. Vaginoplasty is often combined with hymenoplasty.

Labiaplasty

Historically, labial hypertrophy was inconsequential, but now aesthetic and functional concerns are recognized.

In 1655, Armamentarium Chirurgicum had an illustration of clitoral hypertrophy excision by a German surgeon. In 1739, Institutiones Chirugicae, a detailed labiaplasty was described. A simple labiaplasty amputation was done by Radmann in 1976. A detailed description of aesthetic labiaplasty was published in 1983.[4] At that time, the only technique used to reduce the labia minora was the "trim method." However, there were drawbacks like superficial dyspareunia and accentuated clitoral prepuce. In the 1990s, alternative labiaplasty techniques were developed, including the "wedge technique" described by Dr Gary Alter in 1998.[5]

In the 2000s, laser and radiofrequency (RF) techniques improved tissue removal and healing, with "Barbie look" labiaplasty gaining popularity in 2005. By the 2010s, curvilinear labiaplasty and wedge resection became standard, often paired with clitoral hood reduction for balanced aesthetics.

NONSURGICAL PROCEDURES

Platelet-rich Plasma

Over 20 years it has been studied in wound care, orthopedics, dental surgery, spine literature, and a variety of cosmetic surgery procedures.

Marx applied it to mandibular defects in 1998, and its use has since expanded to gynecology and dermatology.

The O-Shot (Orgasm Shot), introduced by Dr Runels in 2011, became a milestone in sexual function enhancement. This procedure involved injecting PRP into areas like the clitoris and vaginal walls to increase sensitivity, lubrication, and overall sexual response. He also used it to treat lichen sclerosus, and introduced the "Vampire Wing Lift".

Today PRP is used for genitourinary syndrome of menopause (GSM), female sexual dysfunction (O-Shot, G-Shot therapy,[6] and lichen sclerosus treatment.

Energy-based Devices

Laser

Laser is an acronym that stands for light amplification by the stimulated emission of radiation, a concept that was developed by Einstein in 1917.

Introduced in 1961, the CO_2 laser gained widespread use in gynecology after Kaplan and colleagues first used it for cervical erosion treatment in 1973, followed by Bellina for cervical intraepithelial neoplasia (CIN) and fallopian tube microsurgery.

In 2010, The MonaLisa Touch, a fractional CO_2 laser, received FDA clearance for treating vulvovaginal atrophy (VVA).[7] The trial of CO_2 lasers in Indian women was done in 2013 in Mumbai, where 35 patients were studied for effects on vaginal tightening and mild to moderate stress urinary incontinence (SUI) .

In the 1990s, the erbium:yttrium-aluminum-garnet (Er:YAG) laser was introduced as a versatile option in cosmetic and gynecological applications, offering precise tissue ablation with less thermal damage. After 2010, the Er:YAG laser became increasingly popular for vaginal rejuvenation and other cosmetic procedures, leveraging its ability to stimulate collagen production while minimizing downtime.

Currently, laser is used to treat dryness, decreased lubrication, dysuria, altered vaginal flora, vaginal laxity, lichen sclerosus in patients in menopause and even in patients after cancer vaginal radiotherapy or systemic hormonal chemotherapy.

Radiofrequency

Initially used for cauterization, RF technology was adapted in 2002 by ThermaCool (SoltaMedical, Inc.) for skin tightening and facial wrinkle treatment after receiving Food and Drug Administration (FDA) approval for its 6-MHz frequency device.

In the 2000s, Dr Red Alinsod began utilizing RF devices in his practice, particularly for vaginal rejuvenation. He played a crucial role in popularizing the use of RF for treating conditions such as vaginal laxity, dryness, and urinary incontinence.[8]

ThermiVa, launched in 2011, gained FDA approval in 2015 for treating vaginal laxity with RF technology.

The first global conversation on RF in aesthetic and functional gynecology was conducted from Mumbai — Indian Academy of Vaginal Aesthetics (IAVA) in 2018, where physicians from across 26 countries participated.

The RF, an energy-based device is currently used to improve genital appearance, sexual function, stress urinary incontinence, lubrication, vaginal laxity, genitopelvic sensation, bowel incontinence, pelvic organ prolapses (POP), and chronic pelvic pain.

A study done on Indian women that included forty-eight patients complaining of sexual dysfunction has shown RF to improve feminine intimate health.[9]

High-intensity Focused Ultrasound

HIFU (high-intensity focused ultrasound) was first investigated for noninvasive ablation in the early 1940s, and in 1994, the first commercial HIFU machine for benign prostatic hyperplasia was launched in Europe; by October 2004, the FDA approved HIFU for treating symptomatic uterine fibroids, and it has since shown promise for placenta accreta, adenomyosis, and endometriosis.

In aesthetic gynecology, HIFU started being used recently, with good study results mostly after 2017. It was shown that intravaginal HIFU therapy results in vaginal tightening, urinary incontinence improvement, and atrophy and genitourinary syndrome treatment.[10]

Electromagnetic Stimulation

In recent years, body shaping has emerged as an increasingly popular and growing area in cosmetic medicine. Magnetic stimulation increases muscle mass and reduces fat volume. High-intensity focused electromagnetic field (HIFEM) and functional magnetic muscle stimulation (FMS) are the common technologies used. HIFEM was approved by the National Medical Products Administration in 2019 to improve the contour of the hip and abdomen.

The electromagnetic field passes in a noninvasive manner and the high frequency of action potentials leads to selective and supramaximal muscle contractions.

The pelvic floor muscles, which are crucial for urinary and bowel control as well as sexual function, were an ideal target for this technology due to their deep location and importance in overall pelvic stability.

A study published in 2020 on a total of 95 patients compared two intervention groups treated with HIFEM (G1) procedure and electrical stimulation (G2), along with the control group (G3), results show that women of age 18–45 years, who had vaginal delivery, have better results using HIFEM.[10] Another study in 2019 included 75 women with symptoms of stress, urge or mixed urinary incontinence, reported a significant reduction of their symptoms using HIFEM treatment.

CONCLUSION

Vaginal rejuvenation procedures are increasing in popularity in terms of types of treatment offered, number of patients undergoing them, clinical studies, and in the controversy surrounding them. Both noninvasive and invasive solutions are being developed by pharmaceutical and technological companies.[11,12]

Today, cosmetic gynecology integrates advanced technologies with a focus on improving quality of life for women, reflecting the dynamic nature of the field and the commitment to patient-centered outcomes.

As gynecologists, understanding this evolution helps to ensure a well-rounded approach to care, combining aesthetic goals with functional health.

REFERENCES

1. Desai SA, Dixit VV. Audit of female genital aesthetic surgery: changing trends in India. J Obstet Gynaecol India. 2018;68:214-20.
2. Goodman MP, Placik OJ, Benson III RH, Miklos JR, Moore RD, Jason RA, et al. A large multicenter outcome study of female genital plastic surgery. J Sex Med. 2010;7(4_Part_1):1565-77.
3. Baskett TF. Eponyms and names in obstetrics and gynaecology. Cambridge University Press; 2019.
4. Chang P, Salisbury MA, Narsete T, Buckspan R, Derrick D, Ersek RA. Vaginal labiaplasty: defense of the simple "clip and snip" and a new classification system. Aesthetic Plast Surg. 2013;37:887-91.
5. Alter GJ, Alter GJ. A new technique for aesthetic labia minora reduction. Ann Plast Surg. 1998;40(3):287-90.
6. Runels C, Melnick H, Debourbon E, Roy L. A pilot study of the effect of localized injections of autologous platelet rich plasma (PRP) for the treatment of female sexual dysfunction. J Women's Health Care. 2014;3(169):2167-0420.
7. Prasad AJ, Pai GS, Pai AH. Laser in aesthetic and regenerative gynecology: physics, types, applications, safety profiles. aesthetic and regenerative gynecology. Singapore: Springer Nature Singapore; 2022. pp . 53-66.
8. Alinsod RM. Transcutaneous temperature-controlled radiofrequency for orgasmic dysfunction. Lasers Surg Med. 2016;48(7):641-5.
9. Desai SA, Vakil Z, Kroumpouzos G. Transcutaneous temperature-controlled radiofrequency treatment: Improvement in female genital appearance, sexual dysfunction, and stress urinary incontinence. Aesthet Surg J. 2021;41(12):1400-8.
10. Bader A, Gynecologist C (Eds). Aesthetic Gynecology Rejuvenation. CRC Press, Taylor & Francis Group; 2024.
11. Desai SA, Kroumpouzos G, Sadick N. Vaginal rejuvenation: From scalpel to wands. Int J Womens Dermatol. 2019;5(2):79-84.
12. Kroumpouzos G, Desai SA, Messas T. Energy-Based Devices for Vulvovaginal Rejuvenation. Adv Cosmetic Surg. 2023;6(1):71-87.

2 CHAPTER

Cosmetic Gynecology: Scope, Evolution and Need

Jaideep Malhotra, Narendra Malhotra, Neharika Malhotra

INTRODUCTION

Cosmetic, aesthetic, and regenerative gynecology are rapidly growing fields that focus on enhancing the appearance, function, and overall quality of life of women. These areas encompass a wide range of procedures, from minimally invasive surgeries to nonsurgical techniques aimed at improving genital aesthetics and addressing functional issues such as sexual dysfunction, urinary incontinence, and postmenopausal changes. This chapter provides an overview of the scope and need for these procedures in modern gynecological practice **(Table 1)**.

Cosmetic gynecology is a rapidly evolving field within gynecology and aesthetic medicine that addresses the aesthetic concerns and functional issues related to the female genitalia. With advancements in medical technology and increasing societal awareness, the scope of cosmetic gynecology has expanded significantly in recent years. Procedures and terminology like "Designer Vagina" 'O' shots, 'P' shots have been commercially patented. Unfortunately, cosmetic gynecology is being commercialized. We need to understand its regenerative and functional more than just aesthetic and cosmetic **(Table 1)**.

Cosmetic gynecology, also known as aesthetic and regenerative gynecology, is a branch of gynecology that focuses on enhancing the appearance and function of the female genitalia. It includes surgical and nonsurgical procedures designed to address both cosmetic and functional concerns in the vulva and vagina.

TABLE 1: Overview of cosmetic, aesthetic, and regenerative gynecology procedures.

Category	*Procedures*	*Purpose*
Cosmetic gynecology	Labiaplasty, vaginal rejuvenation	Enhance aesthetics, improve function
Aesthetic gynecology	Vulvar whitening, G-spot augmentation	Aesthetic enhancement, sexual satisfaction
Regenerative gynecology	PRP, stem cell therapy, exosome therapy	Tissue healing, improved function

Cosmetic Gynecology

- *Vaginal rejuvenation:* Involves tightening of the vaginal canal to enhance sexual function and reduce symptoms of laxity.
- *Labiaplasty:* A surgical procedure to reshape or reduce the size of the labia minora or majora for aesthetic or functional reasons.
- *Clitoral hood reduction:* Reduces excess tissue around the clitoris to improve aesthetics and sexual sensation.
- *Monsplasty:* Reshaping or reduction of the mons pubis area, often combined with liposuction to improve the overall appearance.

Aesthetic Gynecology

- *Vulvar whitening:* Treatments, including laser or chemical peels, to lighten pigmentation for aesthetic enhancement.
- *G-spot augmentation:* Injections to enhance the G-spot area for improved sexual satisfaction.
- *Vaginal resurfacing:* Laser or radiofrequency treatments to improve vaginal mucosa, increase lubrication, and reduce symptoms of vaginal atrophy.

Regenerative Gynecology

- *Platelet-rich plasma (PRP) therapy:* Injections used to promote tissue healing, improve lubrication, and enhance sexual function.
- *Stem cell therapy:* Emerging use of stem cells to regenerate vaginal and vulvar tissues, providing a potential treatment for atrophic changes.
- *Exosome therapy:* Advanced regenerative treatment targeting cellular repair, promoting collagen production, and enhancing tissue health.

EVOLUTION OF COSMETIC GYNECOLOGY: HISTORICAL CONTEXT

The history of cosmetic gynecology traces back to ancient civilizations, where various practices aimed at enhancing female genital aesthetics and function existed. The first references can be seen in Egyptian paintings and in Ratirahasya verse 3 and 4. However, modern cosmetic gynecology as a distinct medical specialty began to emerge in the late 20th century. Initially, procedures were primarily focused on reconstructive surgeries to address congenital anomalies, trauma, or medical conditions affecting the female genitalia.

EMERGENCE AS A SUBSPECIALTY

The late 20th and early 21st centuries witnessed a paradigm shift in cosmetic gynecology, with the introduction of minimally invasive procedures and

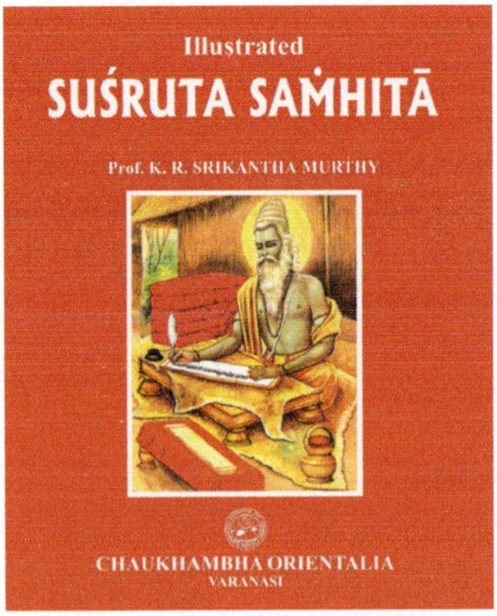

Fig. 1: Sushruta Samhita book.

advancements in surgical techniques and the advent of noninvasive energy base devices. This led to the recognition of cosmetic gynecology as a subspecialty within gynecology and aesthetic medicine. The growing demand for procedures addressing cosmetic concerns such as labiaplasty, vaginal rejuvenation, and clitoral hood reduction further propelled the evolution of this field. Today a lot more indications have been added commonly referred as 'HER Unspoken Problems'. The field of cosmetic gynecology has gained popularity over the years as women seek ways to improve their self-confidence, comfort, and overall well-being. The concept of beauty and aesthetics is not new to our society. In fact, Sushruta, the world's first plastic surgeon, in as early as 600 BC described labiaplasty in his book 'Sushruta Samhita'[1] **(Fig. 1)**. The idea of using warming or heating for rejuvenation, that forms the basis of all energy-based devices (EBD), dates back to centuries when smoke was used to enhance sexual function in women who were newly married, increase vaginal tightness and kill abnormal flora causing infections.[2]

SCOPE OF COSMETIC GYNECOLOGY

Common Cosmetic Gynecology Procedures and their Indications

The cosmetic procedures may be surgical or minimally invasive, nonsurgical procedures that involve EBD. EBD using CO_2 lasers **(Figs. 2A to C),** Erbium YAG laser, Nd:YAG laser, Diode 1470 nm laser **(Fig. 2B)**, low-level laser therapy, radiofrequency **(Fig. 2D)**, high-intensity focused ultrasound (HIFU) **(Fig. 3)**, high-intensity focused electromagnetic waves (HIFEM)

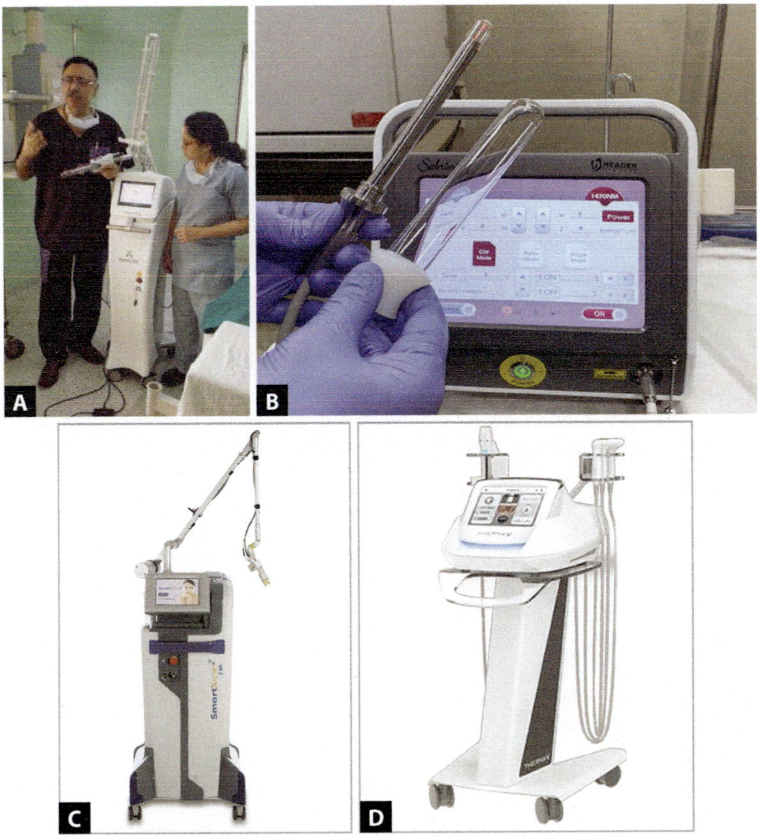

Figs. 2A to D: (A) Femilift CO_2 vaginal probe with guard speculum; (B) Diode 1470 nm laser; (C) MonaLisa Touch laser for vaginal rejuvenation; (D) Radiofrequency probe for vaginal rejuvenation.

(Figs. 4A to C), functional magnetic stimulation **(Fig. 4B)**. These are based on the principle of application of thermal or nonthermal energy to the tissues to cause regeneration, neovascularization, increased epithelial proliferation, to restore physical appearance and function. The various nonsurgical techniques that are used in these procedures are:

- Chemical treatments
- Labial fillers like hyaluronic acid
- Platelet-rich plasma (PRP) (O-shot)
- Carboxy therapy and LED therapy
- Stem cell therapy

Aesthetic (Cosmetic) Procedures

The various aesthetic and regenerative procedures according to their indications can be described in **Table 2**.

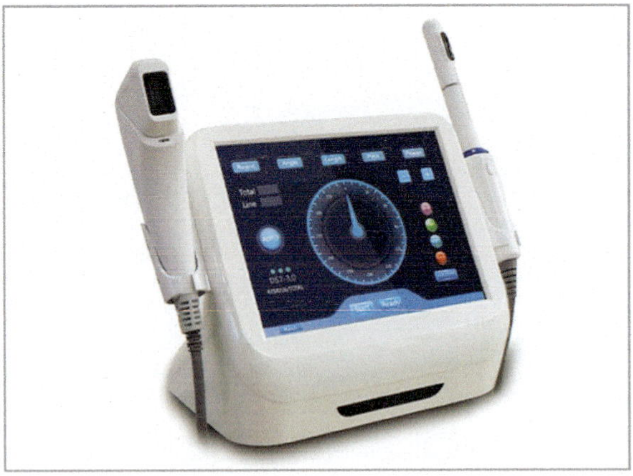

Fig. 3: High-intensity focused ultrasound (HIFU) for skin tightening.

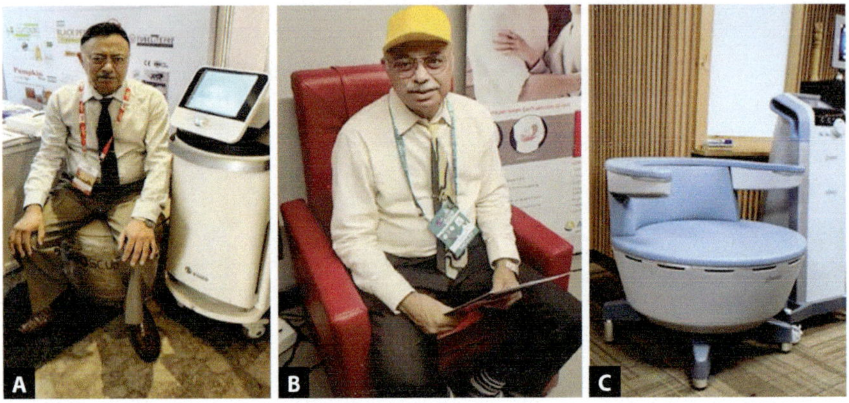

Figs. 4A to C: High-intensity focused electromagnetic waves (HIFEM) chair.

BENEFITS AND CONTROVERSIES

Cosmetic gynecology procedures can offer numerous benefits to women, including improved self-esteem, increased comfort during physical activities, enhanced sexual satisfaction, and relief from functional issues such as urinary incontinence or vaginal laxity. Many women report a significant improvement in their quality of life after undergoing these procedures.[3-6]

However, the field of cosmetic gynecology is not without controversies. Critics argue that some procedures may be driven by societal pressures or unrealistic beauty standards, potentially leading to unnecessary surgeries. Additionally, concerns exist regarding the safety and efficacy of some nonsurgical procedures and the qualifications of practitioners performing these treatments. Further research is needed for the standardization of procedures and results.

TABLE 2: The various aesthetic and regenerative procedures according to their indications.

Cosmetic indications	*Functional indications*
Labiaplasty	Vaginal rejuvenation with radiofrequency for symptomatic relief in vaginal laxity, stress incontinence, enhanced sexual pleasure
Vaginoplasty	Perineal and pelvic musculature strengthen by HIFEM chair
Hymenoplasty	HIFU for vaginal rejuvenation
Monsplasty	Lasers for begnin vulval lesions and diseases
Clitoral hood reduction	PRP and stem cell injections
Noninvasive body contouring	
Carboxy therapy	
G-spot augmentation: Injection of hyaluronic acid or collagen fillers in the female G-spot to improve sexual function	

(HIFEM: high-intensity focused electromagnetic waves; HIFU: high-intensity focused ultrasound; PRP: platelet-rich plasma)

Some major world organizations have tried to address these controversies. In 2015, the International Federation of Gynecology and Obstetrics Committee for the Ethical Aspects of Human Reproduction stated that patients who desire cosmetic gynecologic procedures as well as surgeons must be well versed with the differences between therapeutic and nontherapeutic surgical procedures, the normal anatomy, its function and variations should be explained. Thorough evaluation of the patients should be carried out, especially for body dysmorphic disorders, and the operating surgeons should be competent and trained enough to carry out these procedures.[6]

In 2017, ACOG gave a new committee statement that in cases of patients, especially adolescents who request cosmetic procedures, information must be given to the family members about the procedures, the normal anatomy and their variations, evaluation of the patient's physical and mental state, and choice of noninvasive procedures should be offered.[7]

FDA regulations on energy-based devices: In a July 2018 Safety Communication, the US Food and Drug Administration (FDA) issued a public warning against the use of EBDs in procedures like vaginal rejuvenation or vaginal cosmetic procedures.

It stated that the term "vaginal rejuvenation" is highly 'imprecise' and emphasized that, although the FDA is aware that devices such as lasers are used for a variety of surgical applications, the agency has not approved their use for any specific gynecologic indication.

The vulvovaginal EBD devices in question here include those in use for genitourinary syndrome of menopause (GSM) like laser and radiofrequency (RF) devices.

Concurrent with the FDA's Safety Communication, a December 2018 International Urogynecological Association Writing Group Opinion summarized the small, but growing, body of evidence as well as concerns about vulvovaginal EBD.

An International Continence Society/International Society for the Study of Vulvovaginal Disease Best Practice Consensus Statement published in February of 2019 stated that, based on the currently available literature, it is not recommended to use laser for routine treatment of vulvovaginal atrophy (VVA) or stress urinary incontinence (SUI) except as part of a clinical trial or with special arrangements for clinical governance, consent, and audit.[8]

Female genital mutilation (FGM) is another controversial area and includes procedures that involve partial or total removal, or injury in any form to the female external genitalia for nonmedical reasons. It is a very dangerous practice and causes severe bleeding, urinary problems, infections, as well as complications in delivery and childbirth later in life.

The practice of FGM stems from the gender inequality that is still prevalent in many societies, wherein traditional practitioners carry out these procedures on females and minors as a form of discrimination. It is a violation of the human rights of girls and children. In many scenarios, healthcare providers may be involved in FGM due to the belief that the procedure may be carried out more safely under medical supervision and care. World Health Organization (WHO) strongly prohibits this practice and advises healthcare providers not to perform FGM.[9]

ETHICAL CONSIDERATIONS

Patient Autonomy and Informed Consent

Importance of Informed Consent

Informed consent is a crucial aspect of any medical procedure, including cosmetic gynecology. It is essential for healthcare providers to thoroughly educate their patients about the benefits, risks, and alternatives of each procedure, enabling women to make well-informed decisions about their bodies.

Qualified healthcare professionals must conduct a comprehensive preoperative evaluation to ensure that candidates are suitable for the chosen procedures. They should also take into account the psychological and emotional aspects of the patient's decision, ensuring that expectations are realistic and grounded in healthy motivations.

Both surgical as well as nonsurgical procedures of aesthetic gynecology need due consent before performing. The consent form should have all the details regarding the risks in both cases, purpose of the treatment, procedure, alternatives, success or failure rates.

Ethical considerations are paramount in cosmetic gynecology, particularly concerning patient autonomy and informed consent. Physicians must ensure that patients fully understand the risks, benefits, and potential outcomes of cosmetic procedures, including the implications for sexual function and psychological well-being. Informed consent should be obtained in a comprehensive and empathetic manner, allowing patients to make informed decisions about their care.

Medicalization of Female Genitalia

Critics of cosmetic gynecology raise concerns about the medicalization of female genitalia and the pressure on women to conform to narrow standards of beauty. It is essential for healthcare providers to approach cosmetic procedures with sensitivity and cultural competence, acknowledging the diverse motivations and experiences of patients seeking treatment. Open communication and patient-centered care are essential in addressing these ethical considerations.

FUTURE TRENDS AND CHALLENGES

Technological Advancements

The future of cosmetic gynecology is likely to be shaped by ongoing technological advancements, including the development of minimally invasive techniques, novel surgical instruments, and emerging modalities such as regenerative medicine and tissue engineering. These innovations may offer new possibilities for enhancing both the aesthetic and functional aspects of the female genitalia, with potentially fewer risks and shorter recovery times.

Research and Education

As cosmetic gynecology continues to evolve, there is a growing need for research and education to advance clinical practice and ensure patient safety. Collaborative efforts between gynecologists, aesthetic surgeons, and researchers are essential in establishing evidence-based guidelines, standardized training programs, and best practices for cosmetic procedures. Additionally, increased public awareness and education about the diversity of female anatomy and body positivity are crucial in promoting informed decision-making and reducing stigma surrounding cosmetic interventions.

CONCLUSION

Cosmetic gynecology represents a dynamic and evolving field within gynecology and aesthetic medicine, addressing both aesthetic concerns and functional issues related to the female genitalia. The scope of cosmetic gynecology continues to expand, driven by advancements in medical technology, changing societal norms, and growing patient demand. Ethical considerations regarding patient autonomy, informed consent, and cultural sensitivity are paramount in ensuring the responsible practice of cosmetic procedures. Looking ahead, ongoing research, education, and technological innovation will play key roles in shaping the future of cosmetic gynecology and improving outcomes for patients worldwide.

APPENDIX

InSARG: The only Indian recognized association for Cosmetic Aesthetic Regenerative Gynecology.

What is InSARG?

We are the first organized society of our kind in India, established in 2020. Our mission is to promote advance the field of aesthetic and regenerative gynecology through education, research, and collaboration. Our members are dedicated to providing the quality care to women seeking these treatments. Thank you for visiting our website and learning more about society.

InSARG was founded by a group of esteemed pioneers, including Dr Narendra Malhotra, Dr Ragini Agrawal, Dr Preeti Jindal, and Dr Leela Vyas. The journey began in 2019 with the inaugural international interdisciplinary meet in Chandigarh. This was followed by a significant conference in Agra, where the foundational draft of the society was established, culminating in the cementing of its vision at the Gurugram conference. InSARG aims to unite gynecologists in this innovative field and disseminate knowledge about this revolutionary branch to interested professionals.

REFERENCES

1. Goodman MP, Placik OJ, Benson RH 3rd, Miklos JR, Moore RD, Jason RA, et al. A large multicenter outcome study of female genital plastic surgery. J Sex Med. 2010;7(4 Pt 1):1565-77.
2. Goodman MP. Female cosmetic genital surgery. Obstet Gynecol. 2009;113(1):154-9.
3. Ostrzenski A, Krajewski P, Davis K, Komorowski P, Ostrzenska KM. Postmenopausal female sexual function: is there an "aging effect" on sexual health? Obstet Gynecol Int. 2011;2011:130241.
4. Rouzier R, Louis-Sylvestre C, Paniel BJ, Haddad B. Hypertrophy of labia minora: experience with 163 reductions. Am J Obstet Gynecol. 2000;182(1 Pt 1):35-40.
5. Schellens JH, Ma J, Planting AS, van der Burg ME, van Meerten E, de Boer-Dennert M, Schmitz PI, Stoter G, Verweij J. Relationship between the exposure to cisplatin, DNA-adduct formation in leucocytes and tumour response in patients with solid tumours. Br J Cancer. 1996 Jun;73(12):1569-75.
6. FOGO Committee For The Ethical Aspects Of Human Reproduction And Women's Health. Ethical considerations regarding requests and offering of cosmetic genital surgery. Int J Gynaecol Obstet. 2015;128(1):85-6.
7. American College of Obstetricians and Gynecologists, ACOG Committee Opinion No. 686. Breast and labial surgery in adolescents
8. https://www.contemporaryobgyn.net/view/augs-vaginal-energy-based-devices
9. https://www.who.int/news-room/fact-sheets/detail/female-genital-mutilation

3 CHAPTER

Clinical Anatomy: Perineum, Labia, and Pelvic Floor

Jay Mehta

INTRODUCTION

Understanding of the perineal anatomy is the most important aspect to be studied in cosmetic gynecology. This will help each one of us in doing better procedures and better reconstructions.

LABIA

The labial region is a highly sensitive, region surrounding the external genitalia of the female with a dense network of nerves as well as perforator vessels arising from the pudendal artery which arises from the internal iliac artery. Another supply comes to the mons from the branches of the external iliac artery just below the inguinal ligament.

Labia is divided for categorization into two categories, the labia majora and the labia minora. Both of them arise embryologically from the same compartment. Labia minora is approximating the vaginal orifice. In the same region, we have the external urethral meatus, the anus as well as the clitoris.

The labial region has the presence of a fat pad predominantly for cushioning purposes. This fat pad has a wide variety of applications, which we will discuss later.

PERINEUM

The perineal region is the region between the vaginal orifice and the anus. And predominantly it is a complex which is formed out of many small muscles like superficial and deep transverse perinei, bulbospongiosus muscle, external anal sphincter, the fibers of the levator ani muscle plate **(Fig. 1)**. This is the region which is most commonly affected in cases of perineal tears and injuries, as well as during episiotomy repairs for allowing a vaginal birth. The perineal region also forms an important assessment landmark in the evaluation of pelvic organ prolapse.

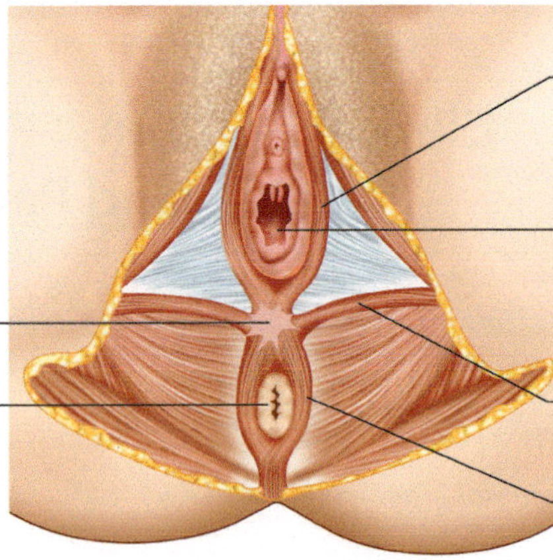

Fig. 1: Anatomy of the perineum.

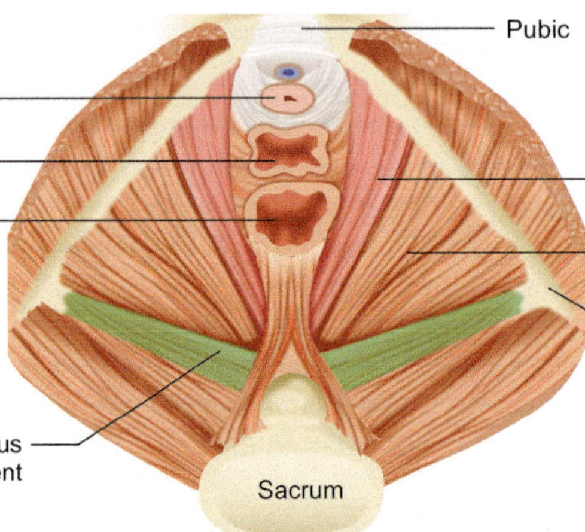

Fig. 2: Anatomy of pelvic floor.

PELVIC FLOOR

The pelvic floor mainly consists of the levator ani muscle plate with all its components, like the pubococcygeus, iliococcygeus and the sacrospinous ligament complex **(Fig. 2)**. The main understanding we need to achieve for this clinical anatomy is that pubovaginalis as well as puborectalis are mainly the fascia surrounding the vagina and the rectum **(Fig. 3)**.

After having discussed this, let's look at the salient points of clinical anatomy we need to know:

- Labia majora and its Fat—can be typically used for martius fat pad which can be mobilized through the perforators of the pudendal artery

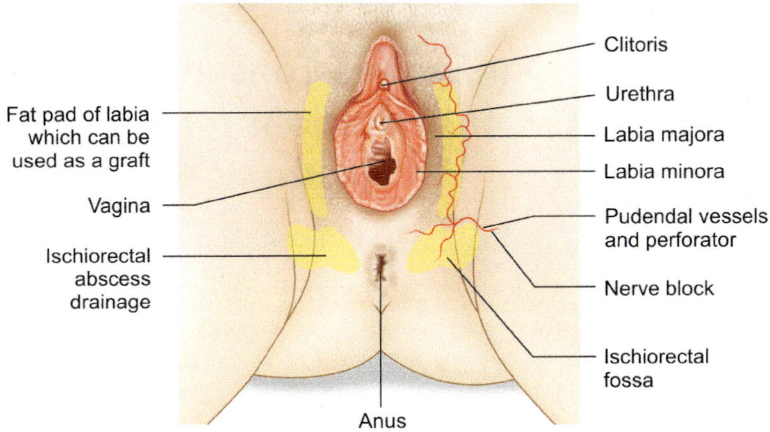

Fig. 3: Anatomy of the labia (applied).

- Labia minora has a common inflammation and involvement in the Bartholin's abscess
- Both the labia can undergo remodeling warranting cosmetic corrections
- Ischiorectal abscess needs a specific drainage
- Lateral wall of the ischiorectal fossa can be used for pudendal blocks
- External sphincter is critical in the repair of the obstetric anal sphincter injury
- Obstetric anal sphincter injury involves a complex repair mechanism and may need a covering ileostomy
- Perineal endometriosis is getting more and more common as an entity
- Perineal body exposure is critical for prolapse repair surgeries
- Hitching the perineal body is not done in prolapse repair as it can cause severe vaginismus
- Vaginismus is mainly due to high tonicity of the bulbospongiosus
- Clitoris and clitoral hood reductions are to be done with endocrinological support

CONCLUSION

This is a chapter to provide an overview. The relevant clinical anatomy varies from patients to patients.

4

CHAPTER

Informed Consent and Legal Considerations for Practice of Aesthetic Gynecology

Parneet Kaur Sekhon

INTRODUCTION

Aesthetic gynecology focuses on procedures aimed at enhancing the appearance and function of female genitalia. Unlike traditional gynecology, which primarily addresses medical concerns related to reproductive health, aesthetic gynecology delves into the realm of elective procedures designed to meet the aesthetic desires and personal preferences of women.[1]

AESTHETIC SURGERY

An aesthetic surgeon is not dealing with a patient with a medical condition, but a healthy individual who wishes for changes in body image. A surgery is not considered cosmetic if there is a documented functional impairment, which may include structural, psychological and/or anatomical concern.[2]

Increased awareness of cosmetic options and a cultural shift towards body image and self-improvement has led to increased demands for aesthetic procedures. For women who present with requests for vaginal cosmetic procedures, a complete medical, sexual and gynecological history must be obtained and the absence of any major sexual or psychological dysfunction including body dysmorphic disorder (BDD) should be ascertained, any possibility of coercion or exploitation must be ruled out.[2]

In responding to a patient's concern about the appearance of her external genitalia, the obstetrician-gynecologist can reassure her that the size, shape and color of external genitalia vary considerably from woman to woman.[3] These variations are further modified by pubertal maturity, aging, anatomic changes associated pregnancy, childbirth and menopause.

CONSENT

Consent means to give an approval, permission and voluntary agreement to a proposition. Informed consent is a fundamental, ethical and legal principle that ensures patients understand the nature of medical procedures, associated risks, benefits, alternatives and potential outcome. The 'adequate information' must be furnished by the doctor (or a member of his team) who treats the patient.

A consent form is not just a signed piece of paper but a document that should include the specifics of the procedure, the expected outcomes, potential complications and side effects and alternative treatment if any. The consent form should be in a language understood by the patient and ensures that she fully understands what she is agreeing to. If required there should be visual aids to help the patient understand the procedure better. The consent of a patient means the participation of the patient in a clinical intervention after achieving an understanding of the relevant medical facts and risks involved.[4]

AESTHETIC SURGERY PROCEDURE

The patient should be of a legal age and mentally competent to give a consent for aesthetic procedures. A minor (<18 years) cannot give consent to a cosmetic procedure. A surgeon must carefully consider psychiatric disorders, including body dysmorphic syndrome, mood disorder, personality disorder, etc.[5] There are strong evidences that patient with BDD does not benefit from cosmetic surgery.[2]

Since aesthetic surgeries are mostly elective, it is the surgeon's legal responsibility not only to take a consent but to make sure the patient has understood the procedure. The cost of the procedure should be discussed with the patient and documented. The local laws should be abided and care should be taken regarding who is eligible to perform the procedure. Patient privacy must be maintained in all aspects. Consent for photographs (if required) should be taken before starting the procedure. Add on procedures not mentioned in the consent form should not be performed and consent cannot be changed during the procedure.

Truthful marketing is a very important legal aspect of aesthetic practice. The rate of claim for procedures should be practical and patient's expectations postprocedure should not be unrealistic. Advertisement in any media must be accurate and not misleading or deceptive.[6]

Complications arising due to a procedure can be tackled if a consent form has been maintained, the patient has been continuously educated to reinforce understanding of the procedure and if no unrealistic expectations were marketed.

CONCLUSION

In conclusion with the advancements in technology, safer and minimally invasive procedures there is an increased willingness among individuals for aesthetic procedures. Aesthetic gynecologists need to respect patient's autonomy while maintaining body positivity. It is not only our legal but ethical responsibility to have an effective communication with our patients to ensure transparency in the procedure.

REFERENCES

1. Gunes A, Allinsod RM. A mini review of aesthetic gynaecology and leading gynaecology associations' approaches to this issue. Turk J Obstet Gynecol. 2018;15:105-11.
2. Shaw D, Allen L, Chan C, Kives S, Popadiuk C, Robertson D, et al. Guideline no. 423: Female genital cosmetic surgery and procedures. J Obstet Gynaecol Can. 2022;44(2):204-14.
3. Elective Female Genital Cosmetic Surgery: ACOG Committee Opinion, Number 795. Obstet Gynecol. 2020;135(1):e36-e42.
4. The American Heritage Medical Dictionary, authors, Houghton Mifflin Company, 2007.
5. Mohindra R. Medical Law Handbook. Radcliff Publishing; 2008. pp. 34-9.
6. ACOG Committee Opinion No. 510: Ethical ways for physicians to market a practice. Obstet Gynecol. 2011;118:1195-7.

5 CHAPTER

Vaginoplasty and Perineoplasty

Sebanti Goswami

INTRODUCTION

Vaginal delivery causes a lot of stretching of the tissues and disruption of the musculofascial attachments in the pelvic floor. Added to this is the atrophy due to menopause and aging. All these insults to the tissues result in gaping of the vagina which lead to decrease in sexual satisfaction and aesthetic concerns. Women may complain of altered sexual satisfaction, reduced friction during intercourse, altered vaginal sensation, and a feeling of laxity. This gaping also creates several functional concerns including excessive vaginal secretions due to mucosa exposure, inability to achieve orgasm, and air entrapment in the vagina causing embarrassing sounds during coitus. Surgical procedures for tightening of the vagina are not new though they have been done historically after delivery. Some studies have shown that surgery for vaginal tightening has resulted in improving the aesthetic quotient and at the same time uplifts the sexual gratification.

The posterior vaginal wall along with the perineum around the fourchette is the target area for this surgery. Vaginoplasty involves tightening of the posterior vaginal wall with the excision of the redundant mucosa whereas perineoplasty narrows the genital hiatus length, removes redundant perineal skin and distal vaginal mucosa, and tightens the introitus with approximation of the superficial transverse perineal and bulbocavernosus muscles.[1] Basically, a surgical technique for vaginoplasty includes introitus and vaginal canal tightening with perineal gap closure and perineoplasty introitus tightening and perineal gap closure. Perineoplasty is specifically indicated for the women who wish to improve the appearance of their perineum postpartum and address their sexual concerns. If a woman complains of dyspareunia, she is not a candidate for perineoplasty.[2]

A complete history should be obtained from the patient including past medical and surgical history (including any prior nonsurgical treatments for vaginal tightening), medications. A gynecological history must also be obtained including: obstetrical history and mode of delivery, history of urinary incontinence, history of hemorrhoids, and any history of any vaginal trauma, sexual dysfunction, sexually transmitted infection, and pelvic malignancy.

Counseling and finding out the exact reason and motivation of the patient for going through this surgery is very important. In many cases, the reason for going under the scalpel is to increase the sexual gratification of the partner. If this is so the woman must be made to understand that there is no surety that this surgery is going to escalate the sexual pleasure of the partner. A thorough physical examination, assessment of the degree of vaginal laxity, the presence of posterior gaping or webbing of the vaginal vestibule, length of the perineal body (i.e., distance between the anus and posterior fourchette), and the presence of hemorrhoids, pelvic mass, pelvic organ prolapse are documented.

PROCEDURE

The procedures are performed under general anesthesia as a day care procedure/local anesthesia with oral or intravenous sedation. Tumescent solution (either epinephrine or vasopressin in normal saline) is injected between the vaginal and rectal mucosa layers to aid hemostasis, while acting as a spacer to protect against an inadvertent rectovaginal fistula.

The surgical markings for posterior vaginoplasty with perineoplasty are designed as two triangular-shaped resection patterns, one internal triangle along the posterior wall of the vaginal canal and one external triangle of the perineum. These two triangles meet at the level of the hymenal ring. This gives an overall diamond-shape excision. The tip of the internal triangle is placed 4–6 cm inferior to the posterior fornix of the vagina. Hymenal remnants are usually identifiable and the medial edge of the two most midline remnants serve as a guide for the width of the planned resection at the level of the hymenal ring. The external marking should transition from the perineal skin to the mucosa of the vaginal vestibule at a right angle.

During a vaginoplasty, the vaginal mucosa is elevated with a combination of sharp and blunt dissection until the levators are exposed. Once the midline mucosa has been split, mucosal flaps are raised laterally in the submucosal plane. Flaps are raised to the level up to which the mucosal resection is planned. The separated edges of the bulbospongiosus muscle are identified and reapproximated using multiple deep interrupted 2-0 Vicryl sutures. The vaginal canal ultimately created should have a diameter of 2.5–3.5 cm and should accommodate approximately two fingers.[1] Overtightening should be avoided as this may result in stenosis of vagina and dyspareunia. In the perineum, the superficial transverse perineal muscles are approximated in the midline. Perineal repair will reconstruct and increase the length of the perineal body, reconstitute the posterior fourchette, and correct posterior gaping of the vaginal vestibule. Overtightening should be prevented to minimize the risk of dyspareunia. Once the muscle repairs have been completed, skin and mucosa are repaired with interrupted 3-0 Vicryl Rapide sutures.

Patients are instructed to take appropriate perineal care for 2 weeks, during which they take antibiotics analgesics and apply ice. Tampons and intercourse are to be avoided for 6–8 weeks.

COMPLICATIONS

Potential complications of vaginal tightening procedures include dyspareunia, vaginal dryness, vaginal and perineal restriction, and rectovaginal fistula. According to one study, the rate of new dyspareunia following posterior colporrhaphy was 15%, with or without levator plication[3] but it might also be due to the reduction of flexibility of the tissues in postmenopausal population. However, much caution is needed to avoid over tightening.

CONCLUSION

Perineoplasty done to address the aesthetic and functional concerns of the vagina is associated with high patient satisfaction rate (around 87.9%), and low complication rates. It is a permanent and relatively easy method of alleviating the sensation of a gaping and loose vagina.

REFERENCES

1. Furnas HJ, Canales FL. Vaginoplasty and perineoplasty. Plast Reconstr Surg Glob Open. 2017;5:e1558.
2. Austin RE, Lista F, Vastis PG, Ahmad J. Posterior vaginoplasty with perineoplasty: a Canadian experience with vaginal tightening surgery. Aesthet Surg J Open Forum. 2019;1(4):1-9.
3. Ulubay M, Keskin U, Fidan U, Ozturk M, Bodur S, Yılmaz A, et al. Safety, efficiency, and outcomes of perineoplasty: treatment of the sensation of the wide vagina. Biomed Res Int; 2016. pp. 2495105. [online] Available from https://www. ncbi. nlm.nih.gov/pmc/articles/PMC5005521/. [Last accessed August, 2017].

6

CHAPTER

Labiaplasty

Parul Saoji

INTRODUCTION

Labiaplasty is shaping the labia to a desired shape and size.

TYPES

- *Labia minoraplasty:* It is shaping the labia minora
- *Labia majoraplasty:* It is shaping of the labia majora
  Labia minoraplasty may also be further classified depending upon the look the patient desires.
  - *Rim:* A natural shape and curve of the labia is maintained
  - *Barbie:* Where the minora are completely dissected
  - *Hybrid:* It is in between the two, where the labia are not too prominent

LABIA MAJORAPLASTY

Shaping of the labia majora is called labia majoraplasty.

Aim

Create youthful appearing majora, which are not excessively protuberant, or not deflated and saggy (common after massive weight loss, aging).

Methods

Surgical Methods

Labia majora reduction surgery is a very useful tool for youthful appearing majora. It can be combined with a labia minoraplasty.

The incision for the surgery is to be taken in the crease so that the scars are not seen. The lateral edges of the incision should be taken such that there is no tension on the suture line and it can be comfortably closed. Under-cutting rather than over-cutting is extremely important. Suture in 3 layers with 4-0 monocryl, after achieving adequate hemostasis.

Minimally Invasive Methods

Autologous fat.

Nonsurgical Methods

- Radiofrequency
- Fillers

LABIA MINORAPLASTY

Shaping up of labia minora is called as labia minoraplasty.

CAUSES OF HYPERTROPHY

- Congenital
- Hormonal
- Myelodysplastic diseases
- Chronic irritation
- Excessive manipulation

INDICATIONS

- Aesthetic
- Intercourse interruption
- Disparity in size
- Unilateral "third labia"
- Stark color difference between the minora and the rest of the pubes.
- Persons who desire to wear tight-fitting clothes, e.g., dancers, horse riders, gym users or persons from the entertainment industry.
- Chronic irritation—chafing by clothes or walking
- Recurrent infections or abscess formation in the minora
- Repairs involving a previous botched procedure.
- Psychological problems like decreased self-esteem, anxiety for intimacy

Exclusion Criteria

- Undiagnosed vulvar lesions, moles or dystrophy
- Active vaginal infections
- *Major medical problems:* It can be done under local anesthesia

CONTRAINDICATIONS

Contraindications include patients with body dysmorphic disorder and those expecting this procedure to enhance their sexual lives and improve their ability to achieve orgasm.

EXAMINATION

Women should always be examined in lithotomy position and with the help of a mirror to show her external genitalia so that she can state her needs.

This also helps in making the patient understand the realistic outcomes of the surgery.

Photographs should also be taken in abducted position. To visualize the projections of labia properly.

METHODS OF LABIA MINORAPLASTY

Labia minora reduction: There is no standard or ideal aesthetic look for labia but by in large few guidelines for labia to look aesthetically appealing are:

- In standing position, the labia minora should not protrude beyond the labia majora
- The clitoral hood should be nonprotruding and short enough without visible folds
- Labia majora should be full but the fat should not be too much and making it look as a bulge in tight clothing
- Also the mons pubis should have the right amount of fat giving it the required fullness but not projecting out of the clothes[1]

  There are three reliable methods for reducing labia minora:

  1. The trim method, also known as the edge method, reported by Hodgkinson
  2. The wedge method pioneered by Alter
  3. Curved linear resection by Alinsod

- *Curved linear resection:* Alinsod's technique includes an incision that starts right below the clitoris, leaving 1 cm of frenulum on either side. The suturing is done in two to three layers with 4-0 or 5-0 monocryl without tension. Avoid dog ears and hide suture lines.
- *Wedge resection:* There can be two types of wedge resections—the anterior wedge or posterior wedge, depending on the labia and the incision preference. The anterior wedge is believed to have a more robust blood supply and healing compared to a posterior wedge. The suturing is done in a similar manner.
- *Trim method:* Asymmetrical labia minora should be corrected with the trim method of excising the excess of labia keeping in mind to leave around 1 cm cuff so that a cover to the introital opening is there.

Advantage for this technique is the operative time is very short and also it creates light-colored labial edges but the same can be problematic for dark skinned patients.

Technique selection should be based on anatomy, patient goals, and patient preferences.[2,3]

COMPLICATIONS OF LABIAPLASTY

Seen in 2.6–6% patients:[4,5]

- Bruising, hematoma
- Infections and wound dehiscence

- Asymmetry, over or under correction
- Dyspareunia, especially if a posterior hammock-like structure created
- Hood Redundancy, or penis like look is common, particularly after curvilinear methods
- Edge dehiscence, fenestrations, scar widening, webbing, pigment mismatch, more common after wedge resections
- Beading of edges
- Fat and fillers—multiple treatments, fat necrosis, embolism
- Majora—scar visibility, vaginal gaping

CLITORAL HOOD REDUCTION

Surgical reduction of the excess clitoral hood skin is often combined with a labia minoraplasty (especially in curvilinear technique) so that the hood does not look very prominent later, giving it a penis like appearance. It is done purely for the aesthetic look, and has nothing to do with improving the intimate sexual experiences. There are two types of hood reductions:

1. Lateral hood reduction
2. Central clitoral hood reduction (CHR)

In both the methods, it is important to stay very superficial to avoid bleeding and injury.

POSTOPERATIVE CARE

When discharging the patient, we need to educate them about the fact they might have severe itching with the dissolution of the sutures.

Also they need to informed of keeping abstinence for 6 weeks. Another thing what they need to take care of is the bowel habits and they should not have any constipation.

Patients are seen after 3 weeks postoperatively to evaluate the healing and also to remove any retained sutures.

CONCLUSION

Labiaplasty is safe and carries a very high rate of satisfaction, though current techniques are very divergent. Key areas for labiaplasty include the anesthesia, resection technique involved and wound closure along with postoperative care.

REFERENCES

1. Alter GJ. Management of the mons pubis and labia majora in the massive weight loss patient. Aesthet Surg J. 2009;29(5):432-42.
2. Clerico C, Lari A, Mojallal A, Boucher F. Anatomy and Aesthetics of the Labia Minora: The Ideal Vulva? Aesthetic Plast Surg. 2017;41(3):714-9.

3. Triana L. Commentary on Anatomy and Aesthetics of the Labia Minora: The Ideal Vulva? Aesthetic Plast Surg. 2017;41(4):993-4.
4. Ouar N, Guillier D, Moris V, Revol M, Francois C, Cristofari S. [Postoperative complications of labia minora reduction. Comparative study between wedge and edge resection]. Ann Chir Plast Esthet. 2017;62(3):219-23.
5. Sharp G, Tiggemann M, Mattiske J. Reply: Psychological Outcomes of Labiaplasty: A Prospective Study. Plast Reconstr Surg. 2017;140(3):507e-508e.

7

CHAPTER

Hymen Reconstruction: Understanding the Procedure and Its Implications

Maalavika Appasani

INTRODUCTION

Hymen reconstruction, also known as hymenoplasty or hymen repair, is gaining attention in various parts of the world especially in countries with conservative cultural views on women's sexuality like the Middle East, Southeast Asia and South Asia. 2018 statistics of India alone shows over 50,000 hymenoplasties on record, reflecting complex interplay of traditional culture and modern healthcare accessibility!

HYMEN BY DEFINITION

It is a thin membranous structure covering the external vaginal opening with most commonly an opening in the center (annual or ring-like hymen) to facilitate menstruation in women.[1]

ROLE OF A HYMEN IN HUMAN BODY

Functionally, there is no use of this membrane in the female reproductive system and also considered remnants of some embryonic tissue.

But historically and culturally in a few parts of the world, its presence signifies purity and virginity in women wherein breaking/tearing of hymen after consummation of marriage bears a lot of importance due to religious, cultural reasons or socio-ethical norms.[2,3]

NEED FOR HYMEN RECONSTRUCTION SURGERY

In this era of women empowerment with debatable moral issues and cultural taboos on considering hymen as a sign of virginity, women are still opting for hymen reconstruction surgeries.[4]

'COUNSELING' A MUST IN ALL CASES

Preoperative counseling allows the woman to make an informed decision to whether to go for the surgery or not. Psychological support pre- and postsurgery is very important in maintaining emotional well-being of the individual and tackling any shame/guilt in facing the society postsurgery.

PROCEDURAL DETAILS

Hymen reconstruction surgery or hymenoplasty is a simple daycare procedure which can be done under local anesthesia or short general anesthesia after a thorough assessment of the patient, where in hymen remnant tissue or a vaginal mucosal flap is taken to create an annular hymen with fine absorbable suture material.

Recovery time is 3–4 weeks for the sutures to be absorbed and sexual intercourse should be avoided during this period. Care should be taken so that the suture site is clean and hygienic to ensure proper healing.[5]

Patients might experience slight pain postoperative which will gradually reduce over a week's time.

LEGAL IMPLICATIONS ON HYMENOPLASTY OR HYMEN RECONSTRUCTION SURGERY

In India, there is no legal regulatory law on hymen reconstruction surgery. So, it is more important to follow medical ethics, bear a clear conscience and informed patient consent.[6]

CONCLUSION

As healthcare providers, it is our duty to approach the practice of hymenoplasty with both medical expertise and cultural sensitivity. It is equally important to spread knowledge and awareness about sexual health and reduce social stigma about virginity by providing proper understanding about women's biology. No matter how big or small the procedure is, surgical expertise with a thorough understanding of anatomy, technique and potential complications is important.

REFERENCES

1. Saraiya HA. Surgical revirgination: Four vaginal mucosal flaps for reconstruction of a hymen. Indian J Plast Surg. 2015;48:192-5.
2. Tschudin S, Schuster S, Dumont dos Santos D, Huang D, Bitzer J, Leeners B. (2013). Restoration of virginity: women's demand and health care providers' response in Switzerland. J Sex Med. 2013;10(9):2334-42.
3. Dhaketa M, Acharya S, Taksande AB, Prasad R, Munjewar PK, Wanjari MB. Hymenoplasty in India: A Comprehensive Review of Contemporary Trends and Impact on Young Adults. Cureus. 2023;15(7):e41852.
4. Christianson M, Eriksson C. Promoting women's human rights: A qualitative analysis of midwives' perceptions about virginity control & hymen 'reconstruction'. Eur J Contracept Reprod Health Care. 2015;20:181-92.
5. Leye E, Ogbe E, Heyerick M. 'Doing hymen reconstruction': an analysis of perceptions and experiences of Flemish gynaecologists. BMC Womens Health. 2018;18(1):91.
6. Mitchell C. The Value of Virginity. J Clin Ethics. 2015;26(2):152.

CHAPTER 8

Labia Majora Augmentation

Purvi Khatri, Krupa Bhagat

INTRODUCTION

Labia majora augmentation is an increasingly popular procedure in cosmetic gynecology, offering both aesthetic and functional benefits to patients. The labia majora, integral to the external genital anatomy, contribute to the appearance and protection of the vulvar region. Factors such as aging, weight loss, hormonal changes, and congenital variations can lead to volume loss, resulting in laxity, discomfort, or dissatisfaction with the appearance of the labia majora.

This chapter explores the anatomy and embryological development of the labia majora, providing a foundation for understanding the procedures aimed at their augmentation. Two primary techniques—autologous fat grafting and dermal filler injections—are discussed in detail, highlighting their indications, contraindications, surgical techniques, and potential complications.

The advancements in labia majora augmentation emphasize patient-centered care, enabling clinicians to address individual concerns while achieving natural, aesthetically pleasing outcomes. Through meticulous evaluation, precise technique, and adherence to safety protocols, these procedures enhance the physical and psychological well-being of patients seeking rejuvenation of the labia majora

ANATOMY

Embryologically, the labia majora in women are derived from genital swellings that, in the male fetus develop into scrotum.[1]

Labia majora are two cutaneous folds that extend posteriorly from mons pubis toward the perineal region. They become wider than labia minora anteriorly and narrow posteriorly.[2] Its outer third has hair bearing and inner aspect lacks hair. Labia majora is filled with subcutaneous fibro fatty tissue to varying degrees, which often is described by patient as 'full' and 'tight' to 'lax' and 'baggy'. Quite commonly lax and baggy appearance as "empty" and "redundant" tissues.

Blood supply of labia majora is from the posterior labial artery and perineal artery, both are branches of the internal pudendal artery. Nerve supply is from the pudendal nerve.

Augmentation of labia majora can be done with the use of autologous fat graft and with the use of fillers.

AUGMENTATION OF LABIA MAJORA WITH AUTOLOGOUS FAT GRAFT

Indications

- Hypoplasia
- Loose skin

  Hypoplasia can be:
  - Congenital
  - Acquired—include
    - Physiological changes in aging and those associated with menopause or during pregnancy
    - Massive weight loss in patients
    - Changes secondary to trauma and tumors
    - Chronic vulvitis

Contraindications

In very thin patients with minimal fat deposition, lack of good donor area is a relative contraindication.

Surgical Technique

Markings

If fat grafting alone is to be performed, then marking should be done in lithotomy position. A long oval-shaped outline is drawn, starting at the level of the outer introitus and extending to the level of pubic prominence (2–3 cm above the distal upper part of the clitoral hood).

Harvesting the Fat Graft

It can be taken from an area where it is available in excess. Inner thigh and abdomen are easily accessed.

Area where liposuction is to be done is marked. Tumescent solution is injected in subcutaneous tissue. Our tumescent solution is prepared using 500 mL normal saline solution, 1 adrenaline ampule (1:1000), and 25 mL of 1% lidocaine.

About 80 to 120 cc of fat may be obtained by liposuction using a 10-mL syringe. 1.8–2 mm cannula is used to extract fat.

Autologous fat graft preparation involves these steps:

- *Fat decantation:* Syringe is placed vertically for 20–30 minutes. Another method is centrifuge it at 1500 rpm for 5 minutes.
- Elimination of liquid, preserving the fat.
- Fat is then transferred from one syringe to another to obtain thinner consistency.

Injecting Fat into Labia Majora

After placing the patient in lithotomy position, an incision is placed on each side of labia majora. Placement of incision should be such that the whole length of labia is treated. If placed too low, then there might be deficiency in the upper aspect fill.

A layered "spaghetti" type approach with injection into deep and superficial layers is essential to prevent necrosis and cyst formation. When fat is introduced, one hand is placed on syringe which softly pushes the syringe embolus, other hand is placed on the marked area guiding the fat to where it needs to stay. At the end of the procedure, fat is molded with both hands.

Result and Outcome

Use of fat injections may achieve the desired outcome,[3] but the integration of fat graft is variable, and some patients may need a secondary procedure to achieve the desired result.[4]

Problems

- Labia majora should have a thinner appearance inferiorly and a wider appearance of the superior aspect. If only fat grafting is performed with loose skin, excess fat should not be placed on the inferior third of labia majora.
- Fat reabsorption can be variable and unpredictable.

Complications

- Fat cyst
- Fat necrosis

Conclusion

Autologous fat graft transfer improves the appearance of vaginal and perineal areas without visible scars and preserves the normal sensitivity to the region.[5]

AUGMENTATION OF LABIA MAJORA WITH FILLERS

- *Main principles of the remodeling or restoration of labia majora with dermal fillers:*
  - Superficial labia majora dermal rejuvenation is similar to rejuvenation of face.

    - Noncross-linked hyaluronic acid is injected intradermal or subcutaneously by needle or cannula.
    - Use of hyaluronic acid along with platelet-rich plasma (PRP) eliminates wrinkles, fine lines and folds.
    - Deep dermal labia majora rejuvenation improves the tone of labia majora providing youthfulness. Depending upon the product used, their effect may stay for 6 months to 1 year.
- *Clinical evaluation and planning:* Patients should use a mirror in lithotomy and standing position so that their concerns could be conveyed properly. Documentation of the anatomy, any variation should be done. The decision of filling the labia should be done after careful assessment and the patient's requirement.

Indications

- Women >18 years of age
- Patients desiring aesthetic rejuvenation of labia majora
- To protect vulva and labia minora in patients with hypotrophy of labia majora.

Contraindications

- Known hypersensitivity to one of the injected components
- Pregnant or breastfeeding women
- Vulvovaginal infections in the injection site (bacterial, viral or fungal)
- Recent vulval surgery in the treatment area or progressive recent or nearby cancers
- Skin inflammation near injection site
- History of autoimmune disease, acute rheumatic fever with cardiac localization or infection with *Streptococcus* disease.

Patient Evaluation

The amount of filler needed should be assessed by comparing and analyzed by thickness of the pubic fat and the protrusion of labia majora.

Preoperative Planning

Antiseptic treatment with intravaginal suppository of neomycin with polymyxin B is started 3 days prior.

Hair clipping is advised 3 days before the procedure.

Surgical Technique

Anesthesia

0.2 mL of xylocaine 2% is injected intradermally on each side. Injection is also to be given subcutaneously along the future path of the cannula.

Markings

Points of introduction depend on the position and preference of operator.

The upper points are in the lateral pubic area, two to three fingers breadth on each side of a vertical center line, between pubis and the posterior commissure. The lower points and the points 2 cm lateral to the labia minora constitute the posterior commissure. The patient is placed in lithotomy position and the surgeon inserts a needle or cannula upwards and diagonally towards the genitocrural furrow. On the proposed cannula pathway, dotted lines are drawn. The direction of the cannula should be oblique, orientation should be toward the perineal node without overflowing inside the free edge of the labia and external remote genitocrural furrow. We stop below the posterior commissure and just above the perineal center.

Materials

- *Needles:* Length 13 mm, 20 mm, 25 mm, diameter 27 gauge to 30 gauge
- *Cannula:* Length 80 mm; diameter 18 gauge
- Xylocaine 2%
- Compresses, gloves
- *Syringes of hyaluronic acid:* 2 mL per syringe
- Sterile pen or markers

Method

After placing the patient in lithotomy position, parts are painted and draped with povidone iodine. A small hole using a 27-gauge needle and a 18-gauge cannula of 8 cm is introduced. The hyaluronic acid filler is injected subcutaneously in retrograde fashion from bottom to top. After the injections, we digitally massage the area for a homogenous distribution of the product.

Postoperative Care

- Patient should not wear tight undergarment for 1 week.
- Not to participate in sexual activity, swimming and sports for a week.

Complications

- Nodule or heterogenous clusters and unsightly labial appearance resembling a pudding or column
- Hematoma
- Cyst
- Painful lymphangitis

CONCLUSION

Labia majora augmentation with filler provides an optimistic result, is safe and a daycare procedure with minimal or no side effects.

REFERENCES

1. Hamori CA. Aesthetic surgery of the female genitalia: labiaplasty and beyond. Plast Reconstr Surg. 2014;134(4):661-73.
2. Triana L, Robledo AM. Aesthetic surgery of female external genitalia. Aesthet Surg J. 2015;35(2):165-77.
3. Triana L, Robledo AM. Refreshing labioplasty techniques for plastic surgeons. Aesthetic Plast Surg. 2012;36:1078-86.
4. Lin JY, Wang C, Pu LL. Can we standardize the techniques for fat grafting? Clin Plast Surg. 2015;42(2):199-208.
5. Vogt PM, Herold C, Rennekampff HO. Autologous fat transplantation for labia majora reconstruction. Aesthetic Plast Surg. 2011;35:913-5.

CHAPTER 9

Complications of Female Cosmetic Gynecological Surgery

Milind R Shah, Naval Shah

INTRODUCTION

Female cosmetic genital surgery (FCGS) has seen a significant rise in popularity in recent years. Procedures like labiaplasty, vaginoplasty, and clitoral hood reduction are sought after by women seeking to enhance the aesthetic and functional aspects of their genitalia. While many women report positive outcomes, it is essential to address the potential complications associated with these surgeries. Understanding the risks involved can lead to more informed decision-making and better patient outcomes. This chapter provides a comprehensive overview of the complications of FCGS, focusing on common issues, psychological effects, long-term consequences, and strategies for risk mitigation.[1]

OVERVIEW OF FEMALE COSMETIC GENITAL SURGERY

Types of Procedures

Female cosmetic genital surgery includes a variety of surgical interventions, each targeting different aspects of the female genitalia. The most common procedures are:

- *Labiaplasty:* Reduces the size of the labia minora or majora to enhance appearance or alleviate discomfort.
- *Vaginoplasty:* Tightens the vaginal canal, often sought after childbirth or for personal reasons.
- *Clitoral hood reduction:* Involves the removal of excess skin covering the clitoris, enhancing aesthetic appearance and possibly sexual pleasure.
- *Perineoplasty:* Repairs and reshapes the perineum, often performed alongside other procedures.

These surgeries can be performed for aesthetic reasons, to address discomfort, or to improve sexual experiences. However, as with any surgical intervention, complications can arise.

COMMON COMPLICATIONS

Infection

Infection is one of the most frequent complications following any surgical procedure, including FCGS. Factors contributing to infection include:

- *Surgical technique:* Poor sterile techniques during surgery can increase infection risk.
- *Postoperative care:* Inadequate hygiene and care can lead to bacterial growth.

Symptoms of infection may include:

- Increased redness and swelling around the surgical site
- Pain that worsens over time
- Pus or abnormal discharge
- Fever and chills.

Management of infections typically involves antibiotics. In severe cases, surgical intervention may be necessary to drain abscesses or remove infected tissue. Preventive measures, such as proper surgical technique and postoperative care instructions, are crucial in minimizing infection risks.[2]

Scarring

Scarring is an inevitable part of the healing process, but abnormal scarring can lead to dissatisfaction. Types of scars include:

- *Hypertrophic scars:* Raised scars that remain within the boundaries of the incision **(Fig. 1A)**.
- *Keloids:* Thick, raised scars that extend beyond the original incision site **(Figs. 1B and C)**.

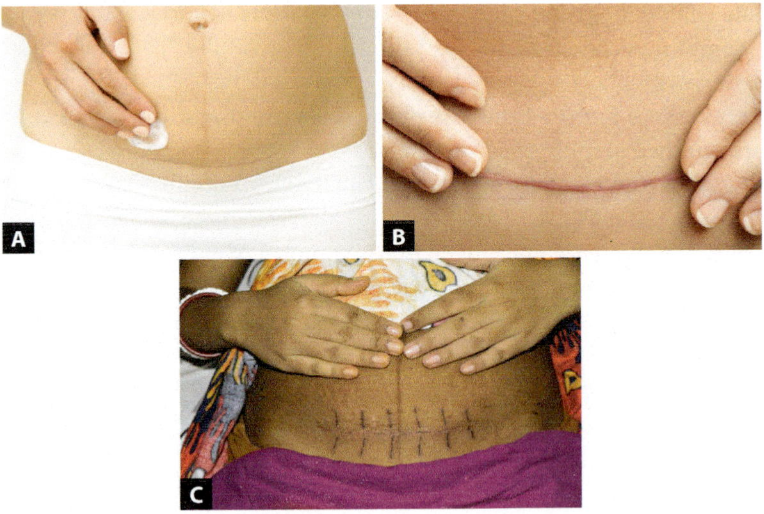

Figs. 1A to C: (A) Hypertrophic scars; (B and C) Keloids.

Management options for problematic scars include:
- *Steroid injections:* Can help flatten raised scars.
- *Laser therapy:* Reduces the appearance of scars.
- *Surgical revision:* In some cases, reoperation may be necessary to improve the aesthetic outcome.

Proper surgical techniques and postoperative care can help minimize scarring. Educating patients about normal healing processes can also set realistic expectations.

Changes in Sensation

Alterations in sensation following FCGS can be a distressing complication for many women. These changes may include:
- *Hyperesthesia:* Increased sensitivity that may lead to discomfort during sexual activity.
- *Hypoesthesia:* Decreased sensitivity, which may diminish sexual pleasure.
- *Numbness:* A total lack of sensation in some areas.

These changes can stem from nerve damage during surgery or excessive scarring. While some women may experience a return to normal sensation over time, others may face long-term issues that impact their sexual health.

Management of sensory changes often involves patient education and counseling. Physical therapy and specialized sexual therapy may also help women adjust to new sensations.

Bleeding and Hematoma Formation

Postoperative bleeding is another potential complication, with hematoma formation being a significant concern **(Fig. 2)**. A hematoma occurs when blood collects outside of blood vessels, leading to:
- *Swelling and bruising:* Noticeable discoloration around the surgical site.
- *Pain:* Increased discomfort in the affected area.

In most cases, small hematomas resolve on their own. However, larger hematomas may require surgical drainage.

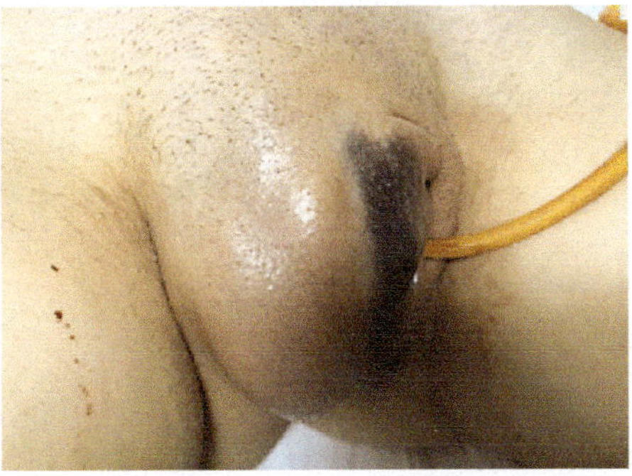

Fig. 2: Postoperative bleeding.

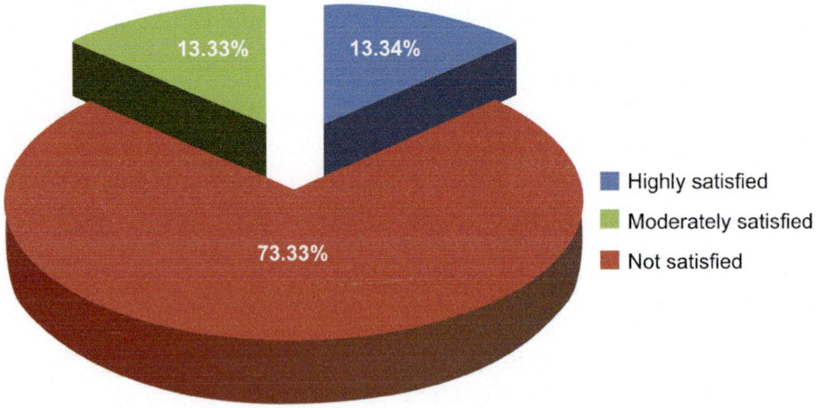

Fig. 3: Level of patient's satisfaction.

Asymmetry and Aesthetic Dissatisfaction

Despite the best efforts of surgeons, aesthetic outcomes can vary significantly. Patients may experience:

- *Asymmetry:* Uneven appearance of the labia or other structures.
- *Overall dissatisfaction:* Not achieving the desired aesthetic or functional result.

Such outcomes can lead to emotional distress and a desire for revision surgery. It is essential for patients to have realistic expectations and for surgeons to provide thorough preoperative counseling regarding potential results.

Psychological Implications

The psychological effects of complications can be profound. Many women may experience **(Fig. 3)**:

- *Anxiety:* Worry about healing, appearance, and future sexual experiences.
- *Depression:* Feelings of disappointment or sadness due to unsatisfactory outcomes.
- *Body image issues:* Concerns about self-esteem and how they perceive their bodies.

Counseling and support groups can be beneficial for women struggling with these psychological challenges. Mental health professionals with experience in body image issues can provide invaluable support and coping strategies.

LONG-TERM COMPLICATIONS

Fistula Formation

Fistulas, or abnormal connections between different bodily structures, can occur in rare cases following surgery. This complication can lead to:

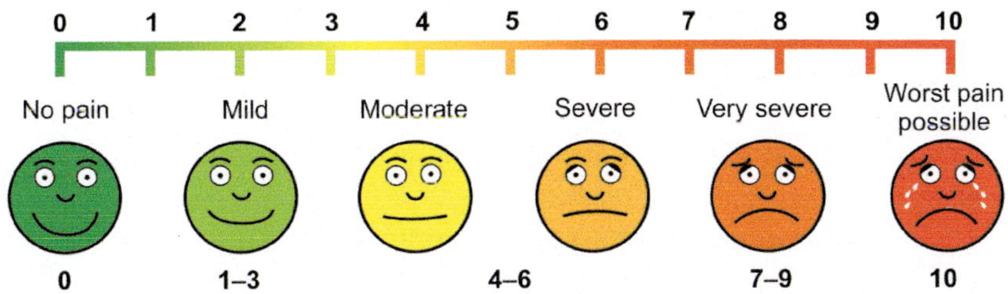

Fig. 4: Pain scale.

- *Chronic discomfort:* Continuous pain or discomfort in the genital area.
- *Infections:* Increased risk of recurrent urinary tract or vaginal infections.
- *Quality of life issues:* Leakage of urine or feces can lead to significant embarrassment and lifestyle changes.

Fistulas often require surgical intervention to correct. Early detection and treatment are critical to minimizing long-term complications.

Chronic Pain

Some women may experience chronic pain postsurgery, which can result from **(Fig. 4)**:

- *Nerve damage:* Injury to nerves during surgical procedures.
- *Scar tissue formation:* Adhesions or tight scars can lead to persistent pain.

Management of chronic pain is multifaceted and may include:

- *Pain management specialists:* Who can provide tailored treatment plans?
- *Physical therapy:* To strengthen pelvic floor muscles and reduce discomfort.
- *Medications:* Such as anti-inflammatories or nerve pain medications.

Reoperation

A significant concern for many women is the possibility of needing reoperation due to complications or dissatisfaction with initial results. Reasons for reoperation can include:

- *Persistent symptoms:* Ongoing pain or discomfort.
- *Aesthetic issues:* Desire for further cosmetic improvement.

While reoperation can provide solutions, it also carries the risks associated with any surgical procedure.

PREVENTION AND MITIGATION STRATEGIES[3]

Choosing a Qualified Surgeon

Selecting a qualified, board-certified surgeon with experience in FCGS is crucial. Researching credentials, reviewing patient testimonials, and assessing surgical outcomes can help ensure that patients receive high-quality care.

Preoperative Assessment

A comprehensive preoperative assessment is vital. This evaluation should include:

- *Medical history:* To identify any pre-existing conditions that may increase risk.
- *Physical examination:* To assess the individual anatomy and discuss specific goals.
- *Discussion of risks:* Providing detailed information about potential complications and outcomes.

Patient Education

Educating patients about the procedures, risks, and expected recovery is essential for setting realistic expectations. Providing detailed preoperative materials and holding questions and answers session can empower patients to make informed choices.

Postoperative Care

Adhering to postoperative care instructions is crucial for minimizing complications. Key aspects include:

- *Hygiene:* Maintaining cleanliness around the surgical site to prevent infections.
- *Monitoring symptoms:* Being vigilant about unusual symptoms and seeking prompt medical attention if they arise.
- *Follow-up appointments:* Regular check-ins with the surgeon to assess healing and address any concerns.

CONCLUSION

While female cosmetic genital surgery can provide significant benefits, it is imperative to understand the potential complications involved. Awareness of these risks empowers women to make informed decisions and advocate for their health. The ongoing evolution of surgical techniques, patient education, and support systems will continue to enhance the safety and satisfaction of women pursuing FCGS.

REFERENCES

1. American Society of Plastic Surgeons. Trends in Cosmetic Surgery; 2022.
2. International Society of Aesthetic Plastic Surgery. Global Statistics; 2022.
3. World Health Organization. Surgical Safety Checklist; 2023.

10A CHAPTER

EBDs: Clinical Uses and Efficacy—Radiofrequency in Aesthetic Gynecology

Deepali Gupta

INTRODUCTION

- Menopause and childbirth are two phases of life which result in many anatomical changes in women life. Previously these women were counseled and made to understand that they need to bear and live with these changes like vaginal laxity, urinary leakage, urge to use washroom very frequently, vaginal pain, dyspareunia, dryness of vagina, recurrent vaginitis and recurrent urinary tract infection (UTI), etc., but with the advent of energy-based devices (EBDs) like radiofrequency (RF) treatment of all these became possible.
- Radiofrequency produces energy in the radio wave range. This energy is used for therapeutic purpose, by changing the physical parameters of RF generator. Normally RF is used to generate endogenous heat in the tissues which, depending on its characteristics, evolves certain therapeutic effects.

WHAT IS RADIOFREQUENCY?

Radiofrequency is a term aimed to describe the oscillation of electromagnetic radiation, meaning the transfer of energy in the form of radio waves, ranging between 3 kHz and 300 GHz.

Radiation can be ionizing or nonionizing. In case of radiofrequency electromagnetic radiation (EMR), it is nonionizing radiation, meaning that it has insufficient energy to break chemical bonds or remove electrons so, this is considered as safe [adopted from ARPANSA (Australian Radiation Protection And Nuclear Safety Agency)].

The RF ranging from 13 MHz to 24 GHz is used to induce heat in a biological tissue, which is turn will respond to accumulated heat and cause cellular and intracellular alterations. There are two mechanisms in which tissue heating may occur, according to the first mechanism, heat is generated due to an ionic current produced by the mobilization of charged particles in an alternating electromagnetic field.

The second mechanism refers to the rotation of water molecules due to an alternating electromagnetic field (3G). In both cases, the particles interaction within the tissues leads to dissipation of energy and volumetric heating of the tissues.

RADIOFREQUENCY: TISSUE INTERACTIONS

Radiofrequency can induce several phenomena on biological tissue:

- *Ablation* is based on exposure of the tissue to high energy density so that tissue is evaporated.[1] As most of the energy is tunneled to ablation, only a small fraction is released as a thermal effect to the margins of the ablated area, yet it is still more substantial than of ablative lasers. RF ablation is commonly used in cautery during surgery.
- *Coagulation* provides hemostasis if blood vessels are present so that bleeding can be controlled during surgery. In ablation, the margins of the evaporated area are coagulated for this purpose. When applied to soft tissue, the coagulative effect induces tissue necrosis without evaporation.[2]
- *Hyperthermia* is heating of the tissue to various temperature levels that do not cause ablation or coagulation. Depending on the temperature reached and the time of exposure, different tissue reaction is seen. Physiological processes that are stimulated include fibroblasts stimulation and collagen synthesis. In cosmetic procedures, the therapeutic temperatures are lowered to avoid epidermal and dermal damage, yet because of the use of lower temperatures, the outcomes may not be consistent, will require multiple sessions and will take longer to show results.

RADIOFREQUENCY DEVICES AND CONFIGURATION

Radiofrequency medical applications are relatively established in fields such as electrosurgery and physiotherapy[3] utilizing tissue heating, commonly referred to as diathermy. RF devices can have different electrode configuration that delivers the current differently **(Fig. 1)**, among them are monopolar, bipolar (multipolar) or unipolar, all have been in use for cutaneous applications.[4] Penetration of monopolar is 20–25 mm, with unipolar 15–20 mm and bipolar reaching approximately 2–8 mm deep.

- Monopolar devices are equipped with a single electrode from which the current is released and a grounding pad to which the current passes. The grounding pad is usually of a large contact area placed outside of the treatment zone so that that high-density RF current is created near the active electrode, and RF current diverges toward the large return electrode.[6]
- Bipolar devices utilize two (or more) closely placed electrodes on the applicator so that current will pass through one to the other while heating a well-defined tissue volume[7] in between the electrodes.

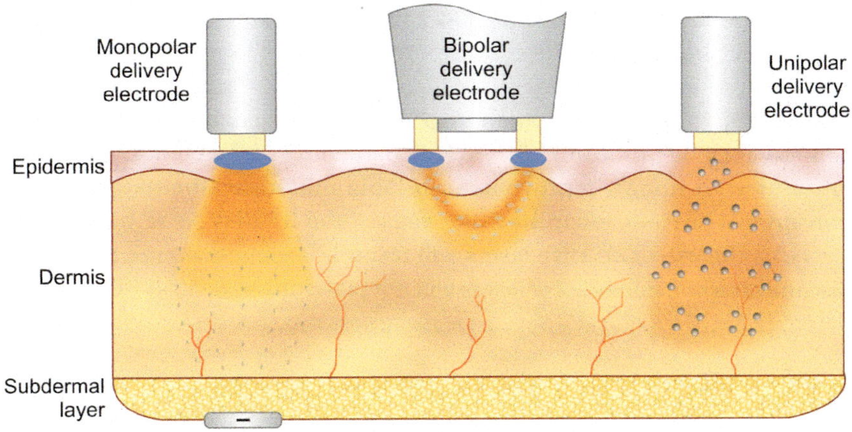

Fig.1: Electroride configurations and heating type on human skin.

- Unipolar current is applied via a single electrode with no need for a grounding pad. It is applied at frequencies higher than 13.58 MHz to create dielectric heating and induce deep tissue penetration, in which maximum heat is located at the central axis of the electrode.[7]

RADIOFREQUENCY IN GYNECOLOGY

Radiofrequency has gained popularity in treating several gynecological procedures during the last years due to its thermal action, based on elevating the temperature of the treated tissue to initiate biological changes. If tissue temperature is quickly elevated beyond a certain threshold, the effect will be of evaporation and ablation of the tissue, yet if the temperature is elevated to lower levels and maintained over a relatively long period of time, a nonablative, the thermal-dependent effect will occur. In gynecology, when applying nonablative RF, the temperature of vaginal wall connective tissue heats up to 40–43°C and generates tightening of the vaginal canal.[8,9] This can be achieved as the heating evokes several biological effects such as inflammation, fibroblasts stimulation, collagen contraction and neocollagenesis. These, in their turn, result in restoration of the vaginal wall, tissue shrinkage and increased moisture of the submucosa.[5,9-11] Early findings also suggest potential neoelastinogenesis, which may contribute to vaginal canal laxity[14] and increased nerve fiber density in papillary dermis which may contribute to improved sexual activity and less emotional distress, lasting a few months postprocedures.[11-13] Other than vaginal laxity, stress urinary incontinence (SUI)[9,14-16] was also explored with promising efficacy and low risk of adverse events in up to 1-year follow-up. Generally, these thermally-related processes are triggered by a nonablative and chromophore-independent mechanism, which makes RF considerably safe regardless to skin type.

Due to moderate nonablative RF also gains the benefit of high comfort and satisfaction during procedures as reported by patients yet associated with significantly longer treatment duration as compared to lasers. In the external genital area, RF was shown to improve aesthetic appearance using ablative and nonablative procedures[16,17] such as tightening of the clitoral hood and introitus with minor improvement in labia minora pigmentation. For a nonsurgical procedure for the outer vagina, the RF may serve better than lasers, as the use of ablative lasers will result in some downtime and slight discomfort while nonablative lasers will not penetrate as deep as RF, thus will probably have less efficacy or require more sessions.[18]

RADIOFREQUENCY TREATMENT PROTOCOL

- No anesthesia required
- The device can exert its therapeutic effect on the skin or mucosa surface at temperature ranging from 39 to 42°C
- Usually, RF device has been embedded safety system to prevent burns
- Frequency used ranging from 1 MHz to 500 Hz to target deep tissues
- Patient feels typically warming sensation at this temperature
- One treatment takes around 20 minutes
- Four treatments are recommended at an interval of 4–6 weeks
- No significant side effects reported
- No downtime, no pain, no discharge

INDICATIONS

Radiofrequency has been shown to be very helpful in treatment

- GSM of menopause
- Vaginal relaxation syndrome after spontaneous delivery
- First and second degree genital prolapse
- Recurrent vaginitis
- Recurrent UTI
- SUI and urge incontinence

REFERENCES

1. Hainer BL. Fundamentals of electrosurgery. J Am Board Fam Pract. 1991;4(6):419-26.
2. Shin MK, Park JM, Lim HK, Choi JH, Baek JH, Kim HJ, et al. Characterization of microthermal zones induced by fractional radiofrequency using reflectance confocal microscopy: a preliminary study. Lasers Surg Med. 2013;45(8):503-8.
3. Mattsson MO, Simkó M. Emerging medical applications based on non-ionizing electromagnetic fields from 0 Hz to 10 THz. Med Dev (Auckland, NZ). 2019;12:347-68.
4. Goats GC. Continuous short-wave (radio-frequency) diathermy. Br J Sports Med. 1989;23(2):123-7.

5. Tadir Y, Gaspar A, Lev-Sagie A, Alexiades M, Alinsod R, Bader A, et al. Light and energy-based therapeutics for genitourinary syndrome of menopause: consensus and controversies. Lasers Surg Med. 2017;49(2):137-59.
6. Duncan D, Kreindel M. Basic radiofrequency: physics and safety and application to aesthetic medicine. In: Lapidoth M, Halachmi S (Eds). Radiofrequency in Cosmetic Dermatology. Basel: Karger Publishers; 2015. pp. 1-22.
7. Lapidoth M, Halachmi S. Radiofrequency in cosmetic dermatology. Aesthet Dermatol. Basel, Karger. 2015;2:50-61.
8. Dillon B, Dmochowski R. Radiofrequency for the treatment of stress urinary incontinence in women. Curr Urol Rep. 2009;10(5):369-74.
9. Karcher C, Sadick N. Vaginal rejuvenation using energy-based devices. Int J Womens Dermatol. 2016;2(3):85-8.
10. Millheiser LS, Pauls RN, Herbst SJ, Chen BH. Radiofrequency treatment of vaginal laxity after vaginal delivery: nonsurgical vaginal tightening. J Sex Med. 2010;7(9):3088-95.
11. Alinsod RM. Transcutaneous temperature controlled radiofrequency for orgasmic dysfunction. Lasers Surg Med. 2016;48(7):641-5.
12. Sekiguchi Y, Utsugisawa Y, Azekosi Y, Kinjo M, Song M, Kubota Y, et al. Laxity of the vaginal introitus after childbirth: nonsurgical outpatient procedure for vaginal tissue restoration and improved sexual satisfaction using low-energy radiofrequency thermal therapy. J Womens Health (Larchmt). 2013;22(9):775-81.
13. Dmochowski RR, Avon M, Ross J, Cooper JM, Kaplan R, Love B, et al. Transvaginal radio frequency treatment of the endopelvic fascia: a prospective evaluation for the treatment of genuine stress urinary incontinence. J Urol. 2003;169(3):1028-32.
14. Leibaschoff G, Izasa PG, Cardona JL, Miklos JR, Moore RD. Transcutaneous temperature controlled radiofrequency (TTCRF) for the treatment of menopausal vaginal/genitourinary symptoms. Surg Technol Int. 2016;29:149-59.
15. Caruth JC. Evaluation of the safety and efficacy of a novel radiofrequency device for vaginal treatment. Surg Technol Int. 2018;32:145-9.
16. Dayan E, Ramirez H, Theodorou S. Radiofrequency treatment of labia minora and majora: a minimally invasive approach to vulva restoration. Plast Reconstr Surg Glob Open. 2020;8(4):e2418.
17. Phenix CP, Togtema M, Pichardo S, Zehbe I, Curiel L. High intensity focused ultrasound technology, its scope and applications in therapy and drug delivery. J Pharm Pharm Sci. 2014;17(1):136-53.
18. Gold M, Andriessen A, Bader A, Alinsod R, French ES, Guerette N, et al. Review and clinical experience exploring evidence, clinical efficacy, and safety regarding nonsurgical treatment of feminine rejuvenation. J Cosmet Dermatol. 2018;17:289-97.

10B CHAPTER

EBDs: Clinical Uses and Efficacy—CO_2 Lasers in Cosmetic Gynecology

Surakshith Battina

INTRODUCTION

Carbon dioxide (CO_2) lasers have emerged as a noninvasive option in cosmetic gynecology, addressing various feminine concerns such as vaginal laxity, vulvovaginal atrophy (VVA), stress urinary incontinence (SUI) and vaginal lubrication issues. These conditions, when considered together, are encompassed under the broader term *genitourinary syndrome of menopause (GSM)*.[1] GSM is a comprehensive term that reflects the multifaceted impact of estrogen deficiency on the genitourinary system. CO_2 laser treatment offers a minimally invasive approach, promoting vaginal tissue regeneration and improving quality of life for women, particularly postmenopausal or postpartum.[2]

MECHANISM OF ACTION

Carbon dioxide lasers emit high-energy infrared light that is absorbed by water within the tissues, leading to controlled thermal damage. This process stimulates collagen production, neovascularization, and the restructuring of the vaginal mucosa. By targeting vaginal tissues, the laser promotes improved elasticity, hydration, and structural support without requiring surgery.[3]

APPLICATIONS IN COSMETIC GYNECOLOGY

Vulvovaginal Atrophy

Vulvovaginal atrophy is a condition affecting postmenopausal women, marked by vaginal dryness, irritation, and painful intercourse. The CO_2 laser helps alleviate these symptoms by promoting tissue regeneration and thickening of the vaginal mucosa. Numerous studies have demonstrated the effectiveness of CO_2 lasers in reducing VVA symptoms and improving vaginal health.[4]

Stress Urinary Incontinence

Stress urinary incontinence occurs due to weakened pelvic floor muscles, often following childbirth or menopause. This condition leads to involuntary urine leakage during physical activities. CO_2 laser therapy strengthens the vaginal walls by stimulating collagen production, which supports the urethra and reduces symptoms of incontinence. Clinical studies have shown improvement in SUI and diaper-free periods after laser treatments.[5]

Vaginal Rejuvenation

Women may seek vaginal rejuvenation procedures to improve both the function and aesthetic appearance of the vaginal area, often due to childbirth or aging. CO_2 lasers cause mild thickening of the vaginal canal by inducing collagen formation, improving vaginal tone and enhancing sexual satisfaction. The defocused laser beam can also be used to apply heat over the vulval area to give it a certain level of "lift" to reduce the skin wrinkling. This nonsurgical method provides functional and cosmetic benefits with minimal downtime.[6]

Improved Lubrication

A significant benefit of CO_2 laser treatments is the improvement in vaginal lubrication. Vaginal dryness, particularly in postmenopausal women or those suffering from VVA, is a major cause of discomfort during sexual intercourse. By stimulating mucosal regeneration and hydration, CO_2 lasers increase natural lubrication, significantly reducing symptoms of dryness.[7]

Enhanced Rejuvenation with Platelet-rich Plasma

An additional benefit of CO_2 laser treatment stems from the microabrasions it creates in the vaginal canal. These controlled microinjuries not only stimulate natural healing and collagen production but also provide an ideal environment for the application of platelet-rich plasma (PRP). When PRP is smeared over the treated area, it enhances the rejuvenation process by promoting faster healing and further stimulating tissue regeneration. This combination therapy leverages the body's natural growth factors to improve overall outcomes in vaginal health and rejuvenation.[8]

EFFICACY AND SAFETY

Carbon dioxide laser treatment for gynecological conditions is generally well-tolerated, with minimal side effects such as mild discomfort, temporary erythema, or slight discharge post-treatment. Patients typically experience significant improvements in vaginal elasticity, moisture, and function following treatment. Clinical trials have demonstrated high levels of patient satisfaction and safety, although long-term data are still being gathered to confirm sustained benefits. Importantly, this therapy serves as a nonhormonal option, appealing to women who cannot or prefer not to use hormone replacement therapy (HRT).

CONTRAINDICATIONS AND CONSIDERATIONS

Though CO_2 laser therapy has demonstrated benefits, it is not appropriate for all patients. Contraindications include active infections, untreated pelvic conditions, and certain medical histories, such as cancerous lesions. A thorough medical evaluation is necessary before initiating treatment. Additionally, patient education is vital to ensure realistic expectations regarding treatment outcomes and the need for potential follow-up sessions.

CONCLUSION

Carbon dioxide laser therapy is a breakthrough in cosmetic gynecology, offering a noninvasive solution for treating a wide range of conditions under the umbrella of GSM, including VVA, SUI, vaginal rejuvenation, and lubrication issues. Its ability to enhance vaginal health, improve sexual function, and restore comfort makes it an attractive option for women, especially those seeking alternatives to hormonal or surgical treatments. With ongoing research, CO_2 laser technology is poised to become a key element in the management of female pelvic health and gynecological wellness.

REFERENCES

1. Baggish MS, Karram MM. Atlas of Pelvic Anatomy and Gynecologic Surgery. Elsevier; 2016.
2. Gambacciani M, Levancini M. Vaginal erbium laser: the second-generation thermotherapy for the genitourinary syndrome of menopause. Climacteric. 2015;18(5):757-63.
3. Salvatore S, Nappi RE, Zerbinati N, Calligaro A, Ferrero S, Origoni M, et al. A 12-week treatment with fractional CO_2 laser treatment of vulvovaginal atrophy: a pilot study. Climacteric. 2014;17(4):363-9.
4. Sokol ER, Karram MM. Use of a novel fractional CO_2 laser for the treatment of genitourinary syndrome of menopause: 1-year outcomes . 2017;24(7):810-4.
5. Gambacciani M, Palacios S. Laser therapy for the restoration of vaginal function. Maturitas. 2017;99:10-15.
6. Gaspar A, Brandi H. Vaginal fractional CO_2 laser for genitourinary syndrome of menopause and stress urinary incontinence: a prospective, observational pilot study. Lasers Surg Med. 2017;49(6):552-9.
7. Filippini M, et al. Efficacy and safety of fractional CO_2 laser treatment in women affected by GSM: A prospective study. Maturitas. 2020;135:48-52.
8. Alinsod R. Noninvasive vaginal rejuvenation and tightening using radio-frequency with or without fractional CO_2 laser. J Minim Invasive Gynecol. 2015;22(1):96-103.

10C CHAPTER

EBDs: Clinical Uses and Efficacy—Erbium Lasers in Aesthetic Gynecology and Regenerative Medicine

Vidya Pancholia

INTRODUCTION AND HISTORY

The aging of tissue generates laxity, and the vaginal mucosa is no exception. Age, vaginal deliveries, weight fluctuations, hormonal changes, instrumentation, and surgeries in the vaginal canal can cause disorders in the vaginal mucosa, producing a sensation of permanent dilation. This can also lead to damage to the pelvic floor which can result in uterine or pelvic organ prolapse and stress urinary incontinence (SUI). Female rejuvenation includes a range of functional and aesthetic procedures in the female genital region. More than half of the female population over age 50 suffers from SUI or some degree of uterine or pelvic organ prolapse. Almost all postmenopausal women have vaginal atrophy, dryness, dyspareunia, and other symptoms associated with menopause.

Vaginal relaxation syndrome (VRS) is a quite common medical condition described as a loss of the optimal vaginal structure and is usually associated with vaginal child delivery and natural aging. Multiple pregnancies and deliveries contribute to a worsening of VRS, as well as the onset of menopause, which causes a decline in hormone levels and vaginal atrophy. VRS results in a decrease or loss of sexual gratification.

The genitourinary syndrome of menopause (GSM) is the new definition for the variety of menopausal symptoms associated with physical changes of the vulva, vagina, and lower urinary tract and is caused by estrogen deficiency. The GSM, caused by estrogen deficiency, is responsible for the appearance of symptoms affecting qualify of life, such as vaginal dryness and/or dyspareunia or urinary symptoms, and affects at least 50% of postmenopausal women.

Female SUI is a highly prevalent lower urinary tract dysfunction, most commonly affecting middle-aged and elderly women. Although the etiology of SUI is not fully understood, the risk factors for the condition include congenital factors, pregnancy, childbirth, hypoestrogenism, cognitive impairment, obesity, and advanced age. Its prevalence has been estimated to be as high as 40% in European countries and 50% in the USA.

There are many possible nonsurgical and surgical therapies for SUI; however, TVT (tension-free vaginal tape), until recently, has been considered as the gold standard in SUI. Initial therapy involves nonsurgical options such as behavioral changes in terms of diet reduction for overweight patients, smoking cessation, bladder training, and pelvic floor muscle training (PFMT). Although good results can be achieved with PFMT, long-term improvement is hard to maintain due to lack of training and poor patient persistence. Mechanical devices such as pessaries, vaginal cones, and urethral obturators and electrical stimulation play an integral part in the management of these patients. Drug therapy also may reduce SUI. Surgical procedures are more effective for SUI than nonsurgical therapies, but are sometimes associated with adverse effects and complications, such as bleeding, bladder perforation, urethral injury, infection, groin pain, and a sexual abstinence period of 6 weeks after surgery. It also has risk of complications of failure of sexual function, discomfort during intercourse, creating excessive obstruction of the lower urinary tract, neuritis of the obturator nerve, and postoperative restrictions. In addition, the recurrence rate for urinary incontinence after surgery ranges from 5.7 to 30–40%.

Noninvasive therapies such as electrical stimulation, radiofrequency, and laser photothermal therapy have been replacing surgical treatment as safer treatment options. Studies have demonstrated collagen remodeling effects of laser irradiation to help strengthen the pelvic floor supportive structures by heating pelvic floor tissue. Many studies have shown erbium:YAG (Er:YAG) laser therapy to be an effective and safe option for different gynecological applications, such as SUI, vaginal relaxation syndrome, and vaginal atrophy (VA).

In terms of evaluating effectiveness of laser procedures, the areas of genital rejuvenation can be broken down into three distinct areas: vaginal atrophy and laxity, SUI, and uterine/pelvic organ prolapse. The laser procedures can further be categorized as follows: noninvasive vs invasive. The only noninvasive laser procedure on the market is a nonablative fractional Er:YAG laser (IntimaLase® and IncontiLase®, Fotona®). All the other laser wavelengths are invasive and include fractional carbon dioxide (CO_2), fractional ablative Er:YAG, and fractional ablative Er:YAG combined with nonablative 1470 diode laser. Devices using radiofrequency are also noninvasive.

One of the first reports on the use of Er:YAG laser technology for gynecological treatments dates back to 2000 when Dr Claudia Pidal and colleagues reported on the use of a Fotona® Fidelis Er:YAG laser (now known as the IntimaLase® and IncontiLase®, Fotona®) for treating vaginal tissue. The results were impressive. The treatment was effective and painless and led to the rapid development of various erbium ablative procedures, including the treatment of human papilloma virus infections, cervical ectropion, vulvar intraepithelial neoplasia, dystrophic lesions, melanosis, and many other conditions. These treatments have also obtained US the Food and Drug Administration (FDA) clearance, and since then thousands of such procedures have been performed in many countries. A high rate of success, with only minor complications, was reported when performing ablation of the lower genital tract, treatment of multifocal and multicentric lesions, excisions, and tissue coagulation. As an interesting and unexpected side effect, many patients reported that they felt a vaginal tightening effect following these Er:YAG treatments, which resulted also in their enhanced sexual experience. This discovery initiated further research in the direction of developing a minimally invasive, nonsurgical, and nonablative erbium treatment for vaginal relaxation syndrome (VRS).

There is a large spectrum of various VRS treatment options on the market ranging from behavioral (Kegel exercises) through pharmacological therapies (hormonal, tightening creams and sprays) to various more or less invasive surgical procedures. While behavioral and pharmacological therapies are noninvasive and safe, they have limited efficacy. On the other hand, various surgical procedures promise a much better final result at the price of higher associated risks. Surgical procedures require the cutting and rearrangement of vaginal and peripheral tissue in order to reduce the size of the vaginal canal. Operating on or near sensitive vaginal tissue is inherently risky and causes scarring, nerve damage, and decreased sensation. Furthermore, patients require an extended recovery period, and the procedure involves considerable pain, discomfort, and risk of infection and serious complications associated with surgery and general anesthesia, including mortality.

Vaginal relaxation syndrome is a quite common medical condition described as a loss of the optimal vaginal structure and is usually associated with vaginal child delivery and natural aging. Multiple pregnancies and deliveries contribute to a worsening of VRS, as well as the onset of menopause, which causes a decline in hormone levels and vaginal atrophy. VRS results in a decrease or loss of sexual gratification. The first studies of the thermal effects of a nonablative Er:YAG on human soft tissue using Fotona® IntimaLase® with SMOOTH mode were performed by Majaron and colleagues in 2000 and Drnovsek and colleagues in 2004. Based on these findings, the nonablative SMOOTH-mode erbium also began to be used on mucosal tissue. The first experiences in targeting mucosal tissue were intraorally. Application of the SMOOTH mode on the soft palate produces tissue contraction, which is an ideal noninvasive method for treating snoring and sleep apnea complications. The first trials with SMOOTH-mode erbium tightening of the vaginal canal had already begun in 2008/2009. Tightening of the vaginal canal and consequently the improvement of sexual gratification were observed.

These trials also revealed that the SMOOTH-mode erbium results in improvement of SUI in women. This resulted in the development of two protocols for two new minimally invasive, nonsurgical, and nonablative procedures: IntimaLase® (for VRS) and IncontiLase® (for SUI). These protocols are based on heating the vaginal wall mucosa up to approximately 65°C and include two treatment sessions with a 4–6-week interval. The time needed to execute the IntimaLase® protocol is approximately 8 minutes and for IncontiLase® around 15 minutes.

The wide use of erbium SMOOTH-mode technology brought further discoveries—in 2013, Bizjack-Ogrinc and Sencar reported excellent results achieved in the reduction of pelvic organ prolapse, and in the same year Gaspar presented his pioneering work on vaginal atrophy. The protocol for treatment of pelvic organ prolapse is based on the sample principle of collagen hyperthermia as are the protocols for vaginal tightening and SUI, although with a difference in the treatment intensity (increased) and the location of the major area treated (the prolapsed part of the vaginal wall). This protocol requires three to five sessions at 4–6-week intervals. The number of sessions is dependent on the severity (grade) of the prolapse. The vaginal atrophy protocol is based on a slightly different concept of milder hyperthermia, whereby the mucosa is warmed up to 45°C, thus causing the stimulation of cell proliferation via heat shock protein activation, an increase of collagen production as well as anti-inflammatory action. This protocol consists of three sessions at intervals of 3 weeks. After immediate tissue shrinkage, the process of neocollagenesis could take up to 6 months to complete.

The vaginal laser received grade I-A level of evidence for improvement of symptoms and tropism for treatment of GSM.

INDICATIONS FOR USE IN GYNECOLOGY (Er:YAG SMOOTH)

General surgery indications: Surgical incision/excision, vaporization and coagulation of soft tissue during any general surgery application, including tissue incision, tissue dissection, excision of lesions, complete or partial resection of internal organs, lesions, tissue ablation and vessel coagulation.

- *Specific gynecology indications:*
    - Herpes simplex
    - Endometrial adhesion
    - Cervical intraepithelial neoplasia (CIN)
    - Cysts and condyloma
    - Stress and mixed urinary incontinence
    - Vaginal relaxation syndrome
    - Vulvovaginal atrophy (VVA)

- GSM
- Pelvic organ prolapse (POP)

- *Genitourinary indications:*
  - Lesions on external genitalia, anus, urethra, scrotum, penis vulva
  - Polyps and familial polyps of the colon
- *Cosmetic indications:*
  - Stretch marks
  - Skin resurfacing ablative and nonablative
  - Skin rejuvenation
  - Treatment of scars—acne, post-trauma, episiotomy
  - Treatment of keloids, warts, skin tags
  - Breast lifting
  - Lip enhancement and refreshing
  - Cheeks enhancement

CONTRAINDICATIONS (Er:YAG)

- Urinary tract infection (UTI)
- Injuries or bleeding in areas of tissue to be treated (vestibule and anterior vaginal wall)
- One of the following urinary tract abnormalities—bladder overcapacity (<300 cc), postvoid residual >50 cc, spastic bladder, vesicoureteral reflux, bladder stones, bladder tumors, urethral stricture and bladder neck contracture
- Abnormal scarring
- Infection or inflammation of treatment area
- Excessive sun exposure (tanned skin)
- A history of a photosensitivity disorder or use of photosensitizing medication
- Pregnancy
- Irradiation in the region of the gonads
- Untreated diabetes

UNDERSTANDING THE SMOOTH® MODE

The SMOOTH® mode of the laser Er:YAG Fotona® (VEL = vaginal erbium laser) is noninvasive **(Fig. 1)** because it acts by pure heating without ablation: it exploits the thermal photo effect of the laser beam on the water present at the mucosal tissue surface. Laser pulses, whose wavelength (2.940 nm) corresponds exactly to the vibratory frequency of the water molecules (3.000 Hz), lead to the rupture of these; this phenomenon generates the synthesis of reactive oxygen derivatives (ROS), which themselves induce a secretion of heat stress (shock) proteins (HSPs) at the origin of the cell repair process. The heat provided to the tissues also causes a contraction of the

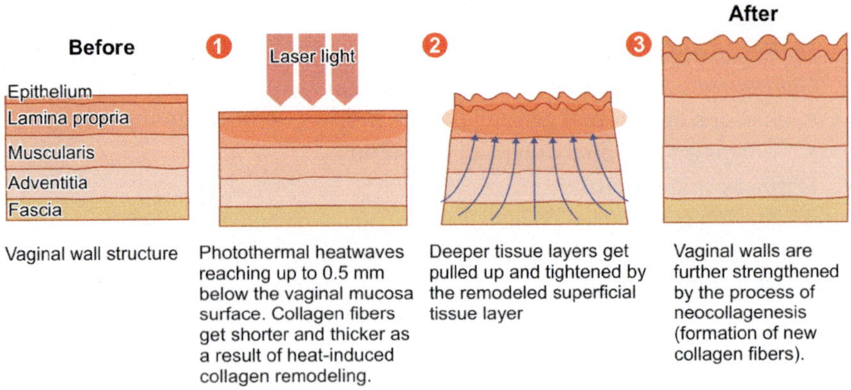

Fig. 1: Action of Er:YAG SMOOTH laser on vaginal tissue.

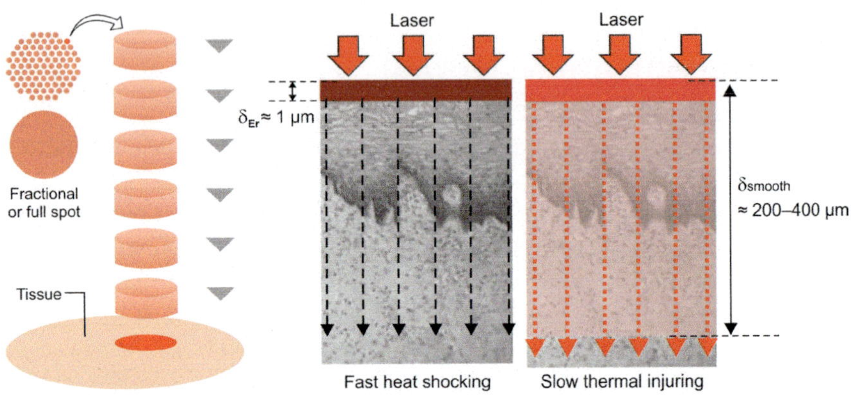

Fig. 2: The process of fast heat shocking of the epithelium + slow thermal stimulation of the connective tissue.

collagen fibers, with fibroblastic stimulation and intense neocollagenesis and angiogenesis. These changes result in an overall improvement in the tone and elasticity of the treated tissue **(Fig. 2)**.

Action 1: Fast heat shocking—effective and safe high temperature heat shock with superficial "triggering" activates a short exposure biochemical process.

Action 2: Slow thermal injuring—involves a long exposure process and "SMOOTH" heating of the deeper lying tissues. Direct slow thermal injury of the connective tissues results in the "conventional" stimulation of fibroblasts.

The thickness of the vaginal mucosa varies but it usually measures several hundred microns. For a controlled deposit of heat at its level, an efficient and safe source of heat is required. SMOOTH® technology is capable of delivering effective stimulating heat over 400 μm in depth without damaging the surface of the mucosa or deeper surrounding tissues. The IntimaLase®,

IncontiLase®, RenovaLase® and ProlapLase® program techniques are based on the nonablative SMOOTH® mode of Fotona®. A SMOOTH® pulse consists of a burst of six low-fluence laser micro-pulses separated by short intervals to refresh the affected surface, thereby avoiding its ablation. Ablation occurs only if the heat brought to the surface is intense and has enough duration: it is the temperature duration of exposure that determines it. The SMOOTH® mode allows a surface temperature of over 250°C to be reached without creating any tissue ablation. Then, the surface heat diffuses toward the depth following a decreasing gradient allowing to obtain the optimal temperature range for neocollagenesis (between 45 and 60°C) up to 400 μm below the mucosal surface **(Figs. 3A to I)**.

It may be noted that this combination of very high temperatures and very short duration is unique to the SMOOTH mode Er:YAG and it sets into action

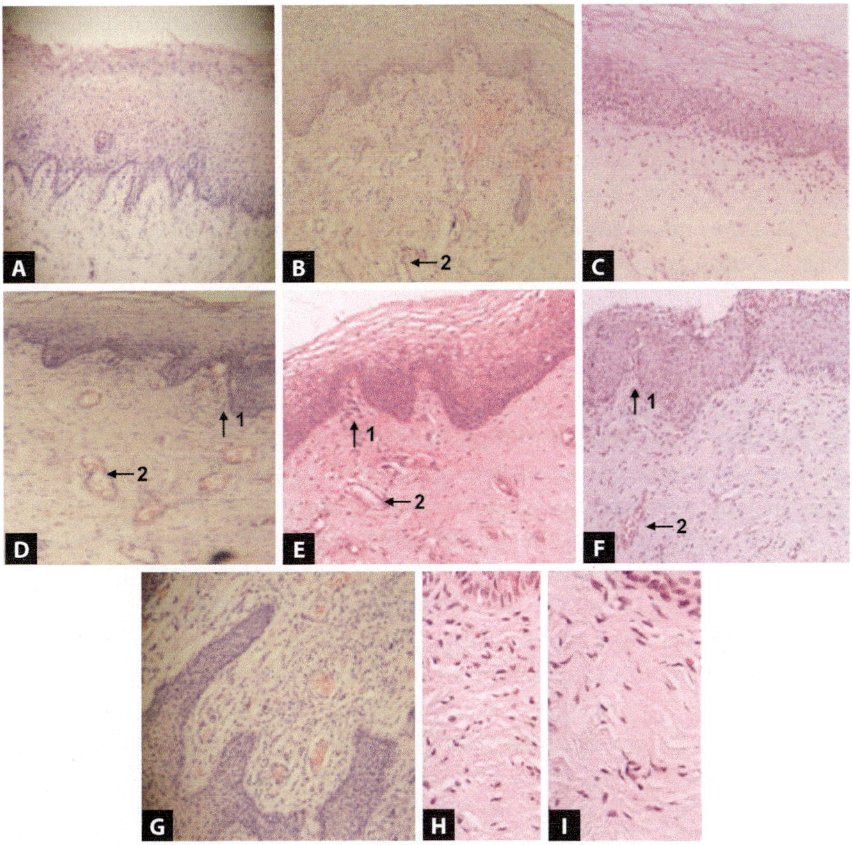

Figs. 3A to I: Vaginal histology before and after Er:YAG SMOOTH Laser VEL.
Source: Gaspar A, Brandi H, Gomez V, Luque D. Efficacy of erbium:YAG laser treatment compared to topical estriol treatment for symptoms of genitourinary syndrome of menopause. Lasers Surg Med. 2017;49:160-8.

the regenerative process by stimulating the Heat Shock Proteins without actual injury. It is only because of the nonablative nature of these pulses that the Er:YAG lasers can be used in both fractional and full beam mode covering 100% of vaginal tissue for a much superior result than any ablative laser whose coverage is limited to only small fraction of the tissue since it causes micro burns and scarring in all the spots that it hits because of the longer duration for which the heat stays on the surface.

HISTOLOGICAL EVIDENCE

Histological examination (hematoxylin-eosin staining) of the vaginal mucosa of patients with GSM symptoms before and after Er:YAG laser treatment. Panel I shows images before treatment **(Fig. 3A)** and at 1 month after laser treatment **(Fig. 3B)**. New vessel formation can be observed. Panel II shows images before treatment **(Fig. 3C)** and at 3, 6 and 12 months after laser treatment [**(Fig. 3D to F)**, respectively]. Increased cellularity and neoangiogenesis can be observed after Er:YAG laser treatment, increase in papillomatosis, basal cells hyperplasia and a complete restorative reaction at the level of the lamina propria. Panel III shows images at 6 months after laser treatment, displaying increased angiogenesis **(Fig. 3G)** and restorative reaction at the level of the extracellular matrix **(Figs. 3H and I)**. Photomicrographs at 4× **(Figs. 3A to G)** and 10× **(Figs. 3H and I)** magnification are presented.

LASER TREATMENT PROCEDURE

The use of the Er:YAG SMOOTH laser for the treatment of SUI. VRS, VA and POP is a novel non-invasive nonablative therapy based on photothermal tightening and shrinking of endopelvic fascia and pelvic floor tissue as well as neogenesis of collagen and angiogenesis which help rejuvenate and improve strength, thickness and health of the treated tissue.

Laser energy from the 2940 nm Er:YAG SMOOTH laser is delivered to the desired locations of the vagina by using specialized handpieces and accessories. A big advantage of Er:YAG is that it can pass through glass and so a reusable glass speculum (shaped like a test tube) is used to completely isolate the patient from coming into contact with the rest of the handpiece and adapters. No anesthesia is required to be administered during the procedure as the patient feels very little discomfort during the treatment (another big advantage of the Er:YAG treatment). The laser handpiece can be either manually inserted into the speculum or a scanner can be used to completely automate the procedure **(Fig. 4)**.

When the laser is activated, it deposits thermal energy in the mucosa tissue of the walls of the vaginal canal covering 100% area with no scarring or burning unlike the ablative CO_2 or ablative Er:YAG which in contrast cover

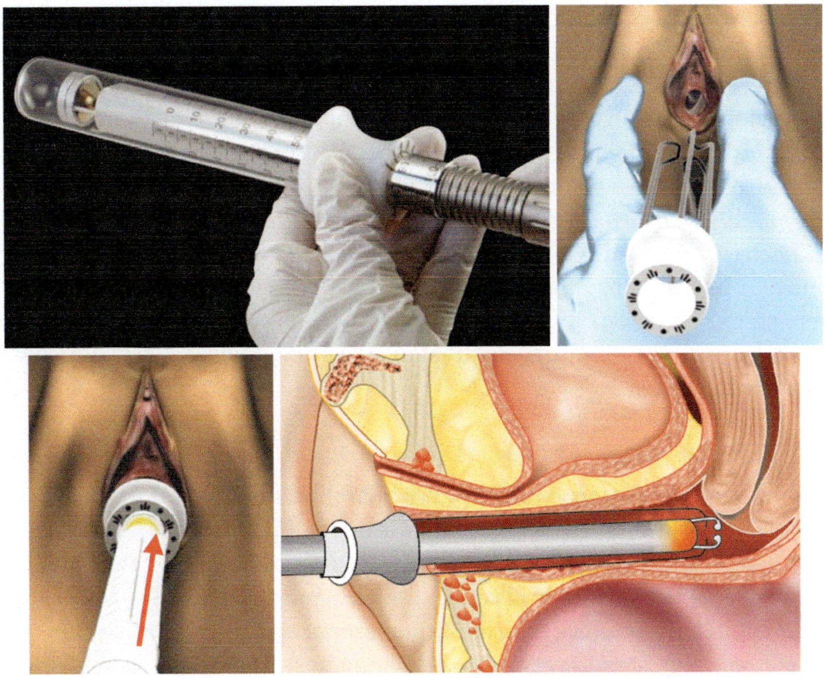

Fig. 4: Glass speculum, inserting speculum into patient, inserting adapter into speculum, laser treatment on the walls of the vaginal canal.

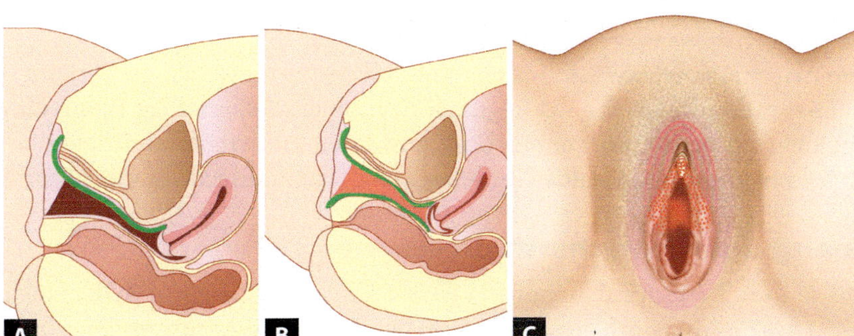

Figs. 5A to C: Selected regions for laser treatment. (A) Anterior wall; (B) Complete walls; (C) External area.

only 5-10% area and cause micro burns. Also, all accessories—everything from the speculum to the hand piece adapters are autoclavable. This means that there are no expensive consumable probes or speculum like with other lasers. This greatly decreases operational expenses **(Figs. 5A to C)**.

The laser is repeatedly activated as the laser beam is gradually moved across the selected vaginal regions (depending on the indication) until the entire area is treated.

Laser therapy for SUI in patients with mild to severe SUI and mixed urinary incontinence (MUI) as well as for treatments up to third degree of POP involves laser shots to all the three regions **(Figs. 5A to C)** and multiple passes depending on severity and patient health.

In the case of vaginal relaxation syndrome or vaginal atrophy, laser shots are only used on two of the three regions **(Figs. 5A to C)** with multiple passes depending on severity and patient health.

Recovery time after an Er:YAG treatment is very short—the patient may return to her daily routine immediately, except that it is recommended to respect standard precautions connected with relapse, such as avoiding efforts which may cause pressure to the treated area or bladder, and to avoid sexual activities for 1 week.

CONCLUSION

There is enough evidence now to show that the nonablative Er:YAG laser is an efficacious and safe new method for the treatment of vaginal laxity, SUI, POP and vaginal atrophy and that it will soon become the treatment of choice for all of these indications and many more. Er:YAG SMOOTH laser treatment is least invasive than any other laser or energy-based treatments or traditional surgical methods for treatment of these indications. It has a much lower complication rate, is well tolerated by patients. Moreover recovery time is very short—the patient may return to daily routine immediately.

ACKNOWLEDGMENT

The material presented in this chapter is based on research carried out in a collaboration with the EU Regional Competency Center for Biomedical Engineering (www.bmecenter.com), and other research coordinated and verified by Laser and Health Academy (www. laserandhealthacademy.com).

Contribution to Authorship

The author, Dr Vidya Pancholia (VP) is a leading Consultant Gynecologist and Laser and Health Academy (LAHA) Expert on Laser application in Gynecology. She conducts LAHA trainings and Laser treatments at her V-Care Laser Clinic in Indore, Madhya Pradesh.

The Co-Author, Mr Krishna Hari (KH) is a Laser Physicist and International LAHA Trainer with over 18 years of experience in the field of laser applications in Aesthetics and Gynecology.

KH instigated the chapter, wrote and edited the manuscript. VP wrote and edited the manuscript. Both authors read and approved the final version of the manuscript

10D CHAPTER

EBDs: Clinical Uses and Efficacy—Diode Laser in Cosmetic Gynecology

AL Satyavati

INTRODUCTION

Since the 1960s, the medical field has witnessed a transformative shift with the advent of laser technology, which has found a wide range of applications across diverse specialties. In the realm of cosmetic gynecology, clinicians have embraced lasers, particularly diode lasers, as a means of revolutionizing cosmetic procedures, offering patients minimally invasive alternatives to traditional surgical techniques that were once the norm.[1]

DIODE LASER: WHAT IS IT?

A *diode* is a semiconductor device that permits electrical current in a single direction. The use of two electrodes achieves this unidirectional flow, hence the name "diode", coined by William Henry Eccles, combining "Di" (meaning two in Greek) and "ode" (short for electrode). While initially used for converting AC to DC (rectification), diodes can also emit light under specific conditions. When electrons jump from a high to a low energy state, energy is released as electromagnetic radiation. When controlled, this release results in a focused beam of directional, monochromatic and coherent source of light known as laser.

MECHANISM OF ACTION

Diode lasers selectively target specific tissues, minimizing damage to surrounding areas. This principle, known as selective photothermolysis, is based on the absorption of near-infrared light emitted by the laser by chromophores like hemoglobin and water within the targeted tissue.[2] This absorption generates heat, leading to precise ablation or coagulation of tissues. Due to better absorption, diode laser wavelengths are particularly well-suited for treating vascular, pigmented, and fibrotic/scarred tissues. They also stimulate collagen production, promoting faster healing and regeneration.

APPLICATIONS OF DIODE LASER IN COSMETIC GYNECOLOGY

In recent times, diode lasers (especially 1470 nm) have emerged as a versatile tool in addressing various cosmetic gynecological concerns.[3] Vaginal atrophy, often associated with menopause, can be effectively treated with diode laser therapy. The treatment stimulates extracellular matrix (mainly collagen) production and improves the elasticity of the vaginal tissue, resulting in enhanced lubrication and reduced discomfort. Other applications include addressing vulvar lesions (benign growths or discoloration), lax vulval folds, labial hypertrophy,[4] mild-moderate stress-urinary incontinence, postdelivery rehabilitation, genitourinary syndrome of menopause (GSM) and postmenopausal symptoms (dryness and recurrent infection).

The healing effects of lasers, which result in the breakdown of old and lax collagen and stimulation of new collagen synthesis, led to the concept of vaginal rejuvenation. More recently, transvaginal and vulvar lasers are being used for several urogynecology conditions such as lichen sclerosis, vulvodynia, overactive bladder, pelvic organ prolapse, etc.

ADVANTAGES AND DISADVANTAGES

Diode lasers offer several advantages, including precise tissue targeting, noninvasiveness, no downtime and high success rate making them popular for clinicians and patients. The 1470 nm wavelength is well regarded for providing controlled heating, while other lasers coagulate and vaporize more tissue leading to pain, downtime and other complications. Moreover, there are new 360° delivery systems that distribute thermal energy to vaginal walls without damaging other tissues, providing better rejuvenation. However, diode lasers may be less effective for treating tissues with a high-water content than other modalities, such as CO_2 or Nd:YAG lasers. Controlling diode laser penetration depth and potential thermal damage requires expertise and careful patient selection.

CONTRAINDICATIONS

Absolute contraindications which prohibit the use of diode lasers include active infections (skin, vaginal, and urinary infection; herpes, etc.), pregnancy, gynecological or oncological pathologies requiring chemo and radiotherapy, and certain medical conditions that increase complication risks. Comprehensive patient assessment, including skin type, medical history, current medications, and any underlying conditions, is crucial to identify potential risk factors and ensure that diode laser procedures are performed on suitable candidates with tailored treatment plans.[5]

PATIENT SELECTION AND EDUCATION

A thorough assessment of the patient's medical history is crucial before considering diode laser procedures in cosmetic gynecology. Clinicians should evaluate the patient's overall physical and mental health as well (for issues like body dysmorphia, which will affect the patient's opinion of postprocedural outcome), including any underlying conditions or medications that might impact treatment safety and efficacy. Information regarding past surgeries, current and past infections, diabetes and other immunosuppressive states, bleeding diathesis (or use of aspirin or similar medication) or other relevant conditions is essential. Importance should also be given to an assessment of the patient's skin type, tone, complexion and keloid tendencies. Obtaining a recent Pap smear report and performing a pregnancy test 1 day before the procedure is also essential. Open communication about potential risks, benefits, expected outcomes, side effects, and postoperative care is vital to ensure the patient's understanding and informed consent. This comprehensive approach enables clinicians to create a tailored treatment plan that maximizes the chances of a successful and safe outcome.

SIDE EFFECTS AND COMPLICATIONS: PREVENTION AND TREATMENT

While generally safe, diode laser procedures can be associated with potential side effects and complications. Patients may experience temporary discomfort, swelling, or redness at the treatment site, which usually resolves with appropriate aftercare and pain management either topically or orally. Hence, it is necessary to inform patients that there may be redness and mild blistering, and the treated area may crust/flake or look like a cat scratch, which will usually last for a few hours and resolve within 14 days, and that each area to be treated usually requires two or more treatments approximately 2–12 weeks apart. Patients should also be informed that even though the lesion may disappear after the procedure, there is still a chance of recurrence, and the fact that it has diminished for several months or years before recurring again suggests that the lesion responded to the treatment and will hence respond in the future as well. However, there are rare but potential risks of infection, bleeding, scarring and even rarer risks, such as injury to surrounding nerves leading to sensory or motor deficits, procedural burn and recurrence of the condition.

Infection: There is a risk of infection at the treatment site, which can be mitigated through proper sterilization of equipment, assessment of patient immunocompetence, adherence to aseptic techniques, and rational use of antibiotics.

Scarring or tissue damage: In rare cases, diode laser treatments may result in scarring or other tissue damage. However, the proclivity for scarring/keloid formation is higher if the patient has a prior keloid tendency.

Pigmentation changes: Diode laser treatments can potentially lead to hyperpigmentation or hypopigmentation in some individuals, particularly those with darker skin tones. It is helpful to rule out any prior dermatological pigmentation disorders, and a dermatologist's opinion can be sought to deal with pigmentation changes.

Blindness/vision loss can occur if the laser is accidentally exposed to the naked eye, so it is mandatory for the patient to wear protective eyewear and close the eyes during the entire laser procedure.

Adjustment of laser parameters and additional laser sessions may also be considered for scarring and pigmentation-related side effects and complications.

By proactively addressing any side effects or complications, clinicians can help minimize the impact on the patient's health and well-being and ensure a positive overall outcome from the diode laser procedure.

FUTURE PROSPECTS

As cosmetic gynecology continues to evolve, diode lasers will likely become increasingly prevalent and refined. Some of the critical areas of future development and advancement in this field may include continued improvement in laser technology with the development of more powerful, precise, and versatile diode laser systems; refinement of treatment protocols and parameters to optimize safety, efficacy, and patient outcomes; expansion of the range of cosmetic gynecological indications that can be effectively treated with diode laser technology, integration of diode laser therapy with other treatment modalities such as radiofrequency or cryotherapy, and increased accessibility and affordability of diode laser technology making it more widely available to healthcare providers and patients.[6]

CONCLUSION

Diode lasers are compact, mobile, easy to use and clean, efficient and relatively inexpensive. They allow for procedures to be done on an outpatient basis, without any cuts or anesthesia. They have a broad spectrum of applications in cosmetic gynecology ranging from vaginal to labial procedures. Despite the proven safety and high efficacy, more research needs to be done to identify newer areas of application with different wavelengths, penetrability and duration of application.

REFERENCES

1. Knappe V, Frank F, Rohde E. Principles of lasers and biophotonic effects. Photomed Laser Surg. 2004;22(5):411-7.
2. Nelson AA, Lask GP. Principles and practice of cutaneous laser and light therapy. Clin Plast Surg. 2011;38(3):427-36.
3. Vitale SG, Saponara S, Sicilia G, Klarić M, Sorrentino F, D'Alterio MN, et al. Hysteroscopic diode laser myolysis: from a case series to literature review of incisionless myolysis techniques for managing heavy menstrual bleeding in premenopausal women. Arch Gynecol Obstet. 2024;309(3):949-59.
4. Zhang R, Wang L. Photodynamic therapy for treatment of usual-type vulvar intraepithelial neoplasia: a case report and literature review. J Int Med Res. 2019;47(8):4019-26.
5. Tian Q, Zhang YX, Wang JJ, Huang GB. Advances in photoelectric therapy for the early intervention and treatment of traumatic scars. Clin Cosmet Investig Dermatol. 2023;16:869-77.
6. Tadir Y, Gaspar A, Lev-Sagie A, Alexiades M, Alinsod R, Bader A, et al. Light and energy-based therapeutics for genitourinary syndrome of menopause: Consensus and controversies. Lasers Surg Med. 2017;49(2):137-59.

10E

CHAPTER

EBDs: Clinical Uses and Efficacy—HIFU (High-intensity Focused Ultrasound)

Manish Mahajan

INTRODUCTION

Vaginal health is an essential component of active and healthy aging in women at midlife and beyond. Quality of life (QoL) would get greatly affected without healthy urological-sexual-genital functions related to vaginal health.

Different physiologic changes in a woman's life such as childbirth, hormonal changes, menopause and ovarian senescence, aging, genetic makeup, weight fluctuations significantly affects anatomy and function of urogenital tissues causing vaginal canal laxity, pelvic floor weakness, mucosal changes. It results into spectrum of symptoms as listed below and the same are *"Indications for energy-based devices (EBDs) use"*:

- Stress urinary incontinence (SUI)—urinary leakage
- Vaginal relaxation syndrome (VRS) vaginal laxity of variable extent
- Feeling of SCOV (something coming out of vagina) without demonstrable prolapse
- Under confidence with changed body appearance
- Poor body image—unattractive feeling
- Genitourinary syndrome of menopause (GSM)—dryness, irritation, burning, itching, easy bruising
- Vaginal dryness causing pain/discomfort
- Dysuria, frequency, urgency
- Recurrent vaginal and urinary infection
- Wrinkles on vulva—slack labia
- Dyspareunia
- Sexuality-related issues—all phases of sexual response cycle are affected causing female sexual dysfunctions.

Various treatment modalities are currently include conservative management with lubricants, HRT, pelvic floor muscle Kegel's exercises and invasive traditional surgical modalities such as anterior repair, posterior repair, colpopexies, colporrhaphy, pelvic floor repair surgeries, Burch colposuspension, mid-urethral sling, meshplasty.

Although these modalities work best with advanced grade of defects, they are insufficient to deal with apparently minor "QoL affecting" complaints. Also, they are associated with risk of surgery—anesthesia, surgical morbidities and complications like mesh erosion.

Treatment advances under fast evolving aesthetic gynecology are helping to fill the lacunae. Cosmetic gynecology is having ongoing advances although most commonly treatment modalities include use of EBDs, regenerative medicine (PRP, stem cells, exosomes, etc.), surgical procedures.

High-intensity focused ultrasound (HIFU) is one of the EBDs used in cosmetic gynecology.

HIFU technique has been popularly and successfully used in cosmetic dermatology and nonsurgical body reshaping since years, use in cosmetic gynecology is simply extension of it.

BASICS AND MECHANISM OF ACTION

As we all know audible acoustic spectrum ranges from 20 to 20 kHz ultrasound starts at 20 kHz.

Imaging involves divergent waves from convex transducer which after reflecting return to form an image that can be used for diagnostic. While HIFU as a therapeutic device has concave transducer where ultrasound waves are convergent to one point generating heat which has therapeutic applications. Similar biophysical principles are used in ultrasound shearers, shockwave lithotripsy, phacoemulsification **(Figs. 1A and B)**.

A round and concave ultrasound transducer of 20 mm in diameter that emits and directs convergent ultrasonic waves. These high-intensity waves focused at a single point at precise focus. Mechanical energy conversion to thermal (60–70°C temperature)/cavitation effect. Resulting in focused

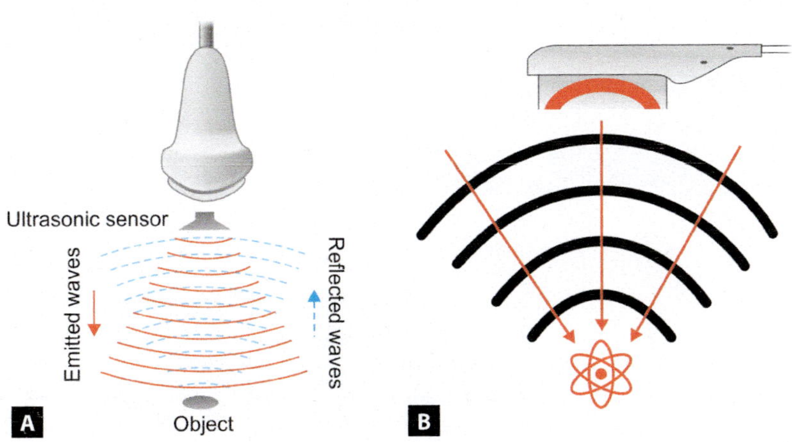

Figs. 1A and B: (A) Convex transducer; (B) Concave transducer.

thermal coagulative microdamage. Controlled regulated heat at one focal point of known depth without burning surface mucosa. Heat produced in 0.1 second lasts for ~3 minutes.

HIFU FOR VULVOVAGINAL REJUVENATION

As most common mechanism of EBDs, HIFU uses biophysical principle of controlled heat-induced collagen remodeling (contraction and firming thereby stimulating neocollagenesis (fibroblast activity), and promoting neovascularization resulting in robust rejuvenation at site of application (vulva as well as vaginal tissue) **(Fig. 2)**.

Commonly two types of vaginal cartridge are commonly available 3 mm and 4.5 mm **(Fig. 3)**. With fixed depth focus point, both cartridge exerts different effects as mentioned below:

- *3 mm head:* Lamina propria—boosts collagen regrowth, improved elasticity, improved vascularity, firming effect

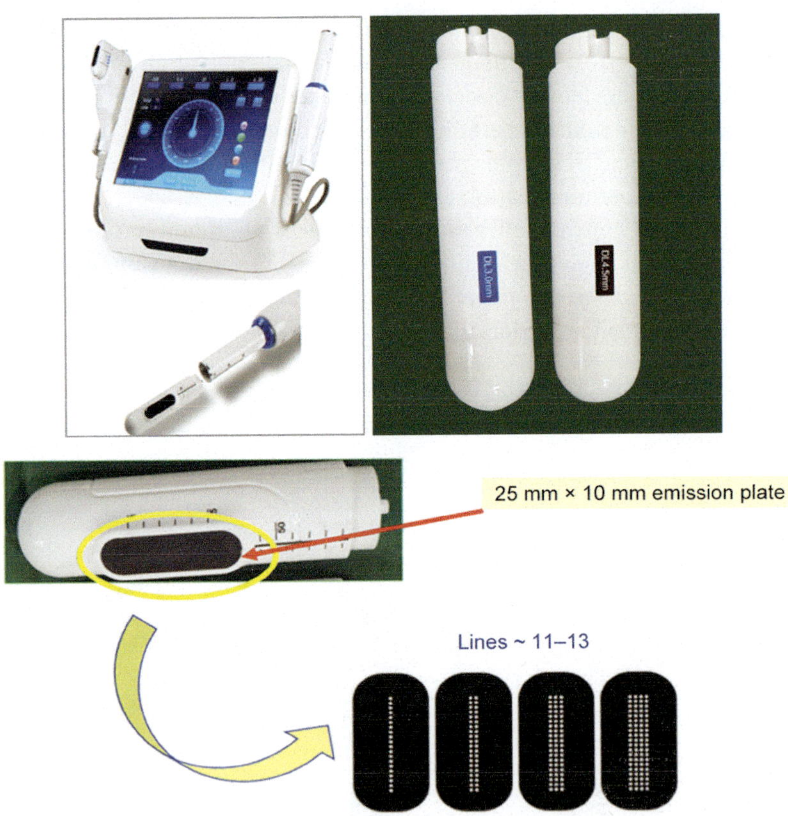

Fig. 2: High-intensity focused ultrasound (HIFU) and its parts.

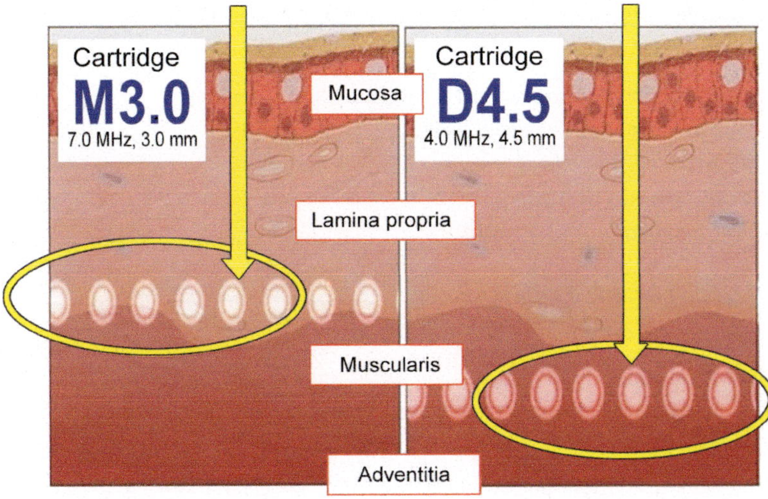

Fig. 3: Vaginal cartridges focus point depth as per different cartridges.

- *4.5 mm head:* Muscularis and adventitial fascial strengthening as well improved elasticity of muscles
- *Superficial 1.5 mm:* Cartridge can be used for vaginal mucosal rejuvenation and vulval skin rejuvenation.

Prerequisite for HIFU Vulvovaginal Application

- Proper patient selection
- Define indication—GSM, LAXITY, SUI
- Detailed medical history
- History of previous such treatments
- Examination
    - SUI, Laxity, POP-Q
    - Rule out pregnancy, malignancy/premalignant lesions
- Counseling and detailed discussion
    - Mechanism of action
    - Desired effects
    - Explain it is a new modality of treatment, although used for specific complaints, it is not yet included as standard treatment modality as compared to the surgical procedures.
    - Variability of outcome including suboptimal OR no result!
    - Possible risks—complications
    - Recurrence of symptoms and need of repeat session
    - Alternative treatment options
- Documentation—written informed consent

Contraindications for HIFU Use in Cosmetic Gynecology

- Pregnancy
- Premalignant conditions and malignancy
- Infection—urinary/vaginal/vulval
- Uncontrolled diabetes
- Chronic steroid therapy
- Advanced urogenital atrophy

ADVANTAGES OF HIFU

- Noninvasive
- OPD Procedure
- Coffee break procedure—treatment sessions last 10–20 minutes
- Easy and safe
- Almost no discomfort other than a warming sensation effective
- Zero downtime with resumption of all activities as normal on the same day, including sexual intercourse
- No anesthesia
- Well tolerated by all patients
- No adverse events or side effects recorded

Additionally, it is useful for wrinkles around eyes, mouth and forehead nonsurgical facelifts—face-tightening, younger looking face with improved collagen, elastin and blood flow, jawline sharpening, for eliminating flaccidity in arms, abdomen and legs, body contouring, etc.

Possible Adverse Outcomes

- Edema and swelling
- Vaginal bleeding
- Vaginitis
- Mild vaginal burn
- Itching
- Burning
- Development of scarring in remote future?

HIFU: VAGINAL REJUVENATION BENEFITS[1,2]

- Improved control over vaginal muscles
- Improved strength of vaginal mucosa
- Improved blood flow
- Improved sensation and sexual pleasure
- Increased resistance to infections
- Correction of mild degree of urinary leakage
- Relief from painful sex due to vaginal causes.

CONCLUSION

Although this is new EBD HIFU in term of vulvovaginal rejuvenation is very effective and safe but as its relatively new, more studies are required to check efficacy as well as reporting any complications.

REFERENCES

1. Elías JA, Galich M, Corin G, Garcia PN, Sivo V, Nestor D, et al. Management of vaginal atrophy, vaginal hyperlaxity and stress urinary incontinence with intravaginal high-intensity focused ultrasound (HIFU) - Int J Obstet Gynecol Res. 2019;6:735-65.
2. dos Santos Borges F, de Carvalho M, de Cerqueira C, Monteiro T, e Benevides I, Dantas A, et al. Vulvar Rejuvenation Using High-Intensity Focused Ultrasound (HIFU): Fundamentals and Technique. Journal of Biosciences and Medicines, 2022;10:239-52. doi: 10.4236/jbm.2022.1012019.

11 CHAPTER

High-intensity Focused Electromagnetic Technology: A Breakthrough, Noninvasive Technology for Treatment of Urinary Incontinence

Preeti Jindal, Ridhi Gulati, Muskan Mittal

INTRODUCTION

Urinary incontinence (UI) is involuntary loss of urine, which objectively and subjectively represents a social, psychological, and hygienic problem. It is estimated that one in every four women aged between 30 and 59 years has experienced a problem with urinary leakage. Estimation of worldwide UI prevalence is around 40% of the female population. However, a vast majority of the patients are reluctant to discuss this intimate issue with their medical doctors. National Association for Continence (NAFC) reports that 4.5 out of 10 patients do not seek help.[1]

Types of urinary incontinence UI can be divided into three types according to its etiology:

1. Clinical symptoms of stress urinary incontinence (SUI) usually involve involuntary leakage of urine when events with increased intra-abdominal pressure are performed (e.g., coughing, sneezing, laughing and lifting). The cause of SUI is due to a loss of support of urethra and deconditioned pelvic floor musculature (PFM), which is usually a consequence of damage to the pelvic support structures. SUI is strongly associated with vaginal childbirth and menopausal hormonal changes.[1]
2. The second UI type is associated with a strong desire to void and pathological contractions of the bladder, so-called urge incontinence. Urge incontinence is a neuromuscular dysfunction commonly treated with pharmacotherapy. Urge incontinence is usually a symptom of an underlying problem (e.g., diabetes mellitus).
3. The third UI type is mixed urinary incontinence (MUI) and involves a combination of the SUI and urge incontinence symptoms.[1]

TREATMENT OPTIONS FOR URINARY INCONTINENCE

The choice of treatment for UI depends on its type and severity. In the case of SUI, treatment options range from noninvasive pelvic floor muscle strengthening from conventional Kegel's exercises to devices like vaginal laser, vaginal high-intensity focused ultrasound (HIFU), vaginal radiofrequency, intraurethral platelet-rich plasma (PRP), intravaginal electrotherapy to surgical intervention. Surgical intervention is recommended usually only in severe cases of SUI, whereas drug treatment of urge incontinence is common. A vast majority of patients use hygienic pads and their quantity depends on the severity of UI and leakage episodes.[2,3]

WHAT IS THE HIFEM CHAIR?

High-intensity focused electromagnetic (HIFEM) chair is a state-of-the-art, noninvasive, painless, and US FDA-approved device used for treatment of pelvic floor muscle weaknesses, UI, and laxity of vaginal muscles. The HIFEM chair helps not only in strengthening and rehabilitating the pelvic floor muscles but also contributes in re-establishing neuromuscular control for treating UI. This device can be used in both males and females.[4]

MECHANISM OF ACTION

High-intensity focused electromagnetic technology triggers intense PFM contractions by targeting neuromuscular tissue and inducing electric currents. Electric currents depolarize neurons resulting in concentric contractions and lift up of all PFMs. Key effectiveness is based on focused electromagnetic energy, in-depth penetration, and stimulation of the entire pelvic floor area. This directly modifies the muscle structure, inducing a more efficient growth of myofibrils—muscle fiber hypertrophy, the creation of new protein strands and muscle fibers—muscle fiber hyperplasia. HIFEM technology causes deep PFM stimulation **(Fig. 1)**.

Supramaximal pelvic floor muscle contractions maximal voluntary contraction (MVC) is the greatest amount of tension that could be developed and held physiologically by the muscle, but usually only for a split second. Contractions with a tension higher than MVC are defined as supramaximal.

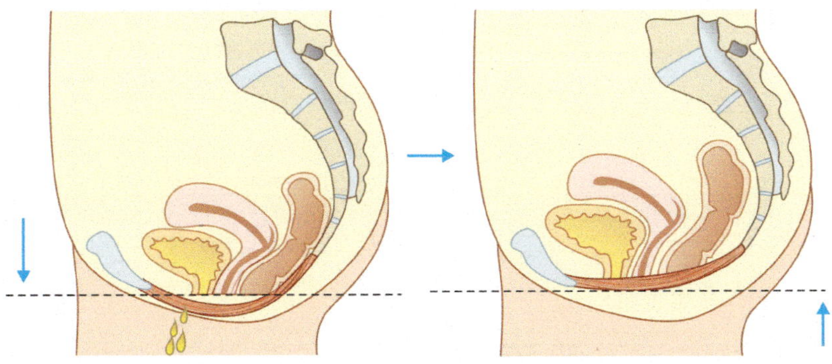

Fig. 1: High-intensity focused electromagnetic (HIFEM) technology causes deep pelvic floor musculature (PFM) stimulation.

HIFEM technology is able to create supramaximal PFM contractions and hold them for a couple of seconds. These contractions are independent of brain function and target directly the peripheral nerves in the pelvic floor area.

Key effectiveness is based on focused electromagnetic energy, in-depth penetration, and stimulation of the entire pelvic floor area. HIFEM technology effectiveness is in the gradually increasing intensity of the focused electromagnetic fields and frequency of pulses, which result in unique vigorousness of the contractions.[1,5-11]

In this device, a coil generates pulsed electromagnetic fields that penetrate deep into the pelvic floor muscles when a person sits on the chair inducing stimulation of the pelvic muscles and contracting them rhythmically in order to strengthen them. The device generates a focused electromagnetic field with intensities of up to 2.5 T and penetration up till depth of 10 cm. The electromagnetic energy produced is directed vertically upward from the center of the seat. The chair design ensures that the patient's perineum is centered when he/she is sitting upright on the chair.[12,13]

This method is extremely important to PFM re-education as the patients are not able to perform this high-repetition rate pattern due to PFM weakness. Such effects cannot be achieved through common exercise (e.g., Kegel) **(Figs. 2 and 3)**.

TREATMENT PROTOCOL

Six sittings are recommended at a frequency of 2–3 sessions per week. Each sitting is a 28-minute treatment session, during which the patient sits in the center of HIFEM chair.

To ensure adequate pelvic floor muscle stimulation, the operator confirms the patient's chair posture throughout the session and adjusts the intensity of stimulus as high as tolerated by patient ranging from 0 to 100.[12]

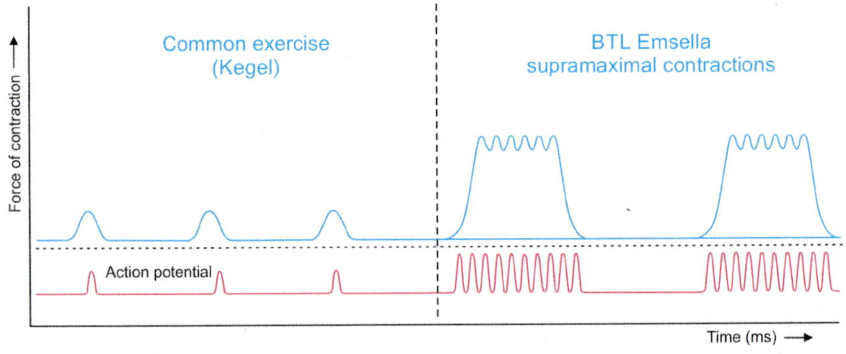

Fig. 2: Pelvic floor musculature (PFM) activation using high-intensity focused electromagnetic (HIFEM) technology compared to common exercises (e.g., Kegel).

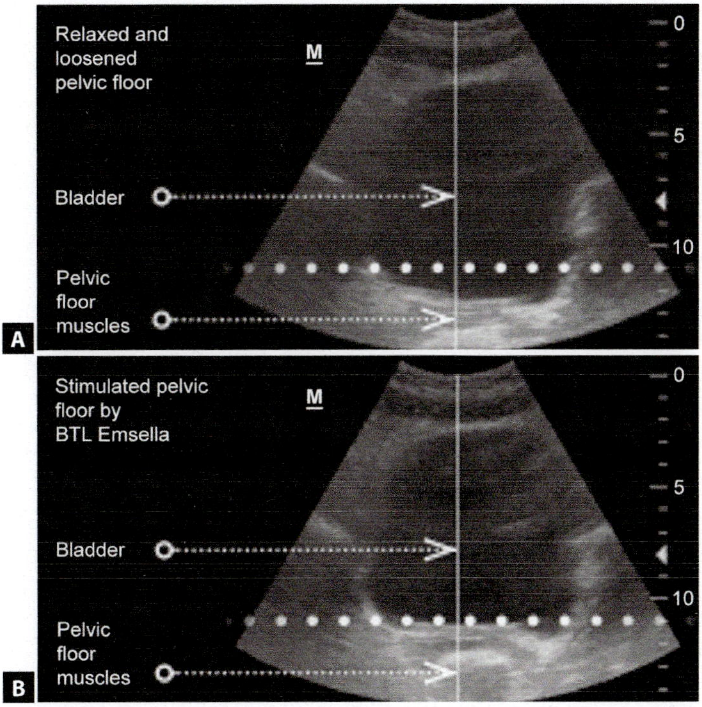

Figs. 3A and B: A frontal view of the pelvic floor muscles and bladder using medical ultrasound. (A) Relaxed and loosened pelvic floor muscles and bladder; (B) Stimulated and lifted pelvic floor muscles and bladder using high-intensity focused electromagnetic (HIFEM) technology.

During this duration, patients may experience contraction and relaxation of muscles throughout the session without any pain.[12] HIFEM chair delivers the equivalent of approximately 11, 200 Kegel exercises in just one session.

INDICATIONS OF USE OF HIFEM CHAIR

- *Stress incontinence:* It is the most common form of incontinence among women and is usually associated with menopause, aging, and/or childbirth. HIFEM chair can help these women with stress incontinence without the risk of infection and complications associated with a surgery as it is noninvasive.[13,14]
- *Sexual rejuvenation:* As HIFEM helps to regenerates and rejuvenates the pelvic floor muscles and vaginal canal, thus in turn it helps to treat sexual dysfunction caused by loss of muscle tone.
- *Urge incontinence:* Urge incontinence occurs when one has a sudden urge to urinate and cannot hold the urine. HIFEM chair can rehabilitate the pelvic floor by contracting and relaxing the muscles of the pelvic floor, thus helping in treatment of urge incontinence.[15]

- *Erectile dysfunction:* HIFEM treatment regulates training of the muscles of the pelvic floor to improve sexual function in males and in turn helps in treatment of erectile dysfunction.
- Pelvic organ prolapse [12]
- Vault prolapse
- Coccydynia

CONTRAINDICATIONS[16] OF USE OF HIFEM CHAIR

- Pregnancy
- Implanted neurostimulators or defibrillators
- Cardiac pacemakers
- Hemorrhagic conditions
- Anticoagulation therapy
- Drug pumps
- Metal implants—hip/knee implants (relative contraindication depending on type implant used)
- Malignant tumors
- Copper-T
- Heart disorders
- Fever

PRECAUTIONS

- Patients should dress comfortably (preferably light fabric bottoms without zippers) on the treatment days.
- Patients should take off jewelry.
- Patients should not wear jeans or thick clothing.
- One should take out credit cards and coins from the pockets.
- Patients should take out iPads, watches, or phones as electromagnetic energy may harm the devices.

ADVANTAGES

- It is painless, noninvasive, and safe 28-minute OPD treatment procedure
- No recovery or healing time involved
- One may remain fully clothed during the treatment
- Significant improvements after a single session
- FDA approved

CONCLUSION

HIFEM chair is a completely noninvasive and safe procedure. A single session lasts for about 28 minutes and most of the patients experience improvements after six sessions.

During the treatment, patients stay fully clothed. Usually, there is no pain associated with the HIFEM treatment and there is no requirement of anesthetics. Patients can resume normal activities on a daily basis immediately after the HIFEM treatment.

REFERENCES

1. Abrams P, Blaivas JG, Stanton SL, Andersen JT. The standardisation of terminology of lower urinary tract function. The International Continence Society Committee on Standardisation of Terminology. Scand J Urol Nephrol Suppl. 1998;114:5-19.
2. Wallis M, Davies E, Thalib L, Griffiths S. Pelvic static magnetic stimulation to control urinary incontinence in older women: a randomized controlled trial. Clin Med Res. 2012;10(1):7-14.
3. Yamanishi T, Yasuda K, Sakakibara R, T Hattori, H Ito, S Murakami. Pelvic floor electrical stimulation in the treatment of stress incontinence: an investigational study and a placebo controlled double- blind trial. J Urol. 1997;158:2127-31.
4. Haylen BT, DeRidder D, Freeman RM, Swift SE, Berghmans B, Lee J, et al. An International Urogynecological Association (IUGA)/International Continence Society (ICS) joint report on the terminology for female pelvic floor dysfunction. Int Urogynecol J. 2010;21(1):5-26.
5. Almeida FG, Bruschini H, Srougi M. Urodynamic and clinical evaluation of 91 female patients with urinary incontinence treated with perineal magnetic stimulation: 1-year follow-up. J Urol. 2004; 171(4):1571-4.
6. Bickford R, Guidi M, Fortesque P, Swenson M. Magnetic stimulation of human peripheral nerve and brain. Neurosurgery. 1987;20(1):110-6.
7. Coletti D, Teodori L, Albertini M, Rocchi M, Pristerà A, Fini M, et al. Static magnetic fields enhance skeletal muscle differentiation in vitro by improving myoblast alignment. Cytometry A. 2007;71(10):846-56.
8. Ishikawa N, Suda S, Sasaki T, Yamanishi T, Hosaka H, Yasuda K, et al. Development of a non-invasive treatment system for urinary incontinence using a functional continuous magnetic stimulator (FCMS). Med Biol Eng Comput. 1998;36(6):704-10.
9. Ostrovidov S, Hosseini V, Ahadian S, Fujie T, Parthiban S, Ramalingam M, et al. Skeletal muscle tissue engineering: methods to form skeletal myotubes and their applications. Tissue Eng Part B Rev. 2014;20(5):403-36.
10. Stölting M, Arnold A, Haralampieva D, Handschin C, Sulser T, Eberli D. Magnetic stimulation supports muscle and nerve regeneration after trauma in mice. Muscle Nerve. 2016;53(4):598-607.
11. Wallis M, Davies E, Thalib L, Griffiths S. pelvic static magnetic stimulation to control urinary incontinence in older women: a randomized controlled trial. Clin Med Res. 2012;10(1):7-14.
12. Jindal P, Sahdev S, Gulati R, Kundal I. Nonsurgical management of stress urinary incontinence (SUI). Acta Sci Women's Health. 2020;21:15-4.
13. Samuels JB, Pezzela A, Berenholz J, Alinsod R. Safety and efficacy of a non-invasive high- intensity focused electromagnetic field (HIFEM) device for treatment of urinary incontinence and enhancement of quality of life. Lasers Surg Med. 2019;5(10):760-6.

14. Jindal P, Gupta M, Isha K. Female urinary incontinence-are visit on prevalence of this problem in todays society, which is increasing due to increase in average life span. Acta Scientific Womens Health. 2021;39:27-33.
15. Swift S, Ostergard D. Sex hormones and the female urinary tract. Int Urogynecol J. 1993;42:32-6.
16. Deshpande J, Singh CK. Emsella: A breakthrough, noninvasive technology for treatment of incontinence. Indian J Obstet Gynecol Res. 2023;05:28.

12

CHAPTER

Carboxytherapy

Preeti Jindal, Pragati Tandon, Muskan Mittal

INTRODUCTION

Carboxytherapy originated in France in the 1930s, where it was used to treat peripheral vascular diseases. Since then, its applications have expanded into various fields, particularly aesthetic medicine. The procedure entails the controlled infusion of medical-grade CO_2 gas into the skin or subcutaneous tissues, with the aim of enhancing circulation and promoting tissue regeneration due to reverse *Bohr effect*. The treatment has been found to stimulate lipolysis (fat breakdown), improve skin elasticity, and reduce the appearance of wrinkles and scars. In 2008, carboxytherapy was found to produce collagen synthesis.[1] There is also the mechanical undermining by the gas flow similarly like in needle subcision (e.g., in the treatment of scars, adhesions or severe cellulite depressions). There are effects of mechanical tension on the cells (especially in rejuvenation) and pressure (especially in the treatment of cellulite or adiposities) resulting from relatively strong gas flow during the CO_2 administration. Presumably there is also some slight influence of temporary acidosis.[2,3] When injected intradermal, thickening of the dermis and rearrangement of collagenous fibers is shown to be increasing skin elasticity. Changes are probably due to improved microcirculation and oxygenation of the tissue.[4] This effect leads to tightening the skin and decreasing flaccidity. Therefore, intradermal and subcutaneous administration of CO_2 (carboxytherapy) is being used as a medical noninvasive or minimally invasive treatment for many inaesthetic conditions.[6] Carboxytherapy is a safe procedure and is a good alternative in the removal and treatment of various skin and subdermal defects and inaesthetics.[5] CO_2 is drained into the blood vessels and eliminated by the lungs; while a little portion is converted into carbonic acid and is eliminated through the kidneys.[6]

TREATMENT

Required material **(Figs. 1A and B)**:

- CO_2 machine which will warm the medical category CO_2 and deliver it under required preset target organ appropriate pressure

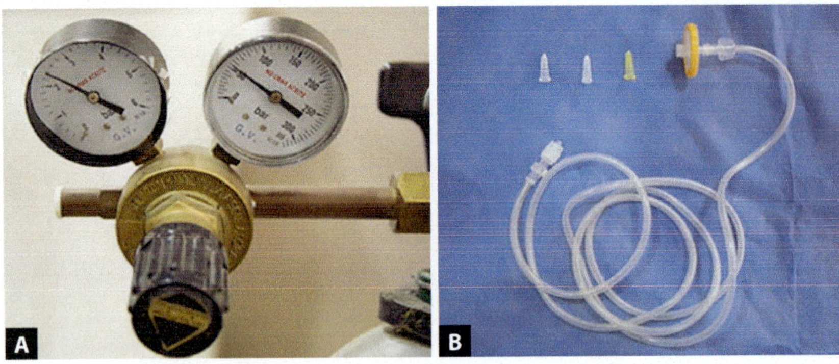

Figs.1A and B: (A) Gas flow regulator; (B) Particle filter and sterile tube for injection. 30 G (yellow)1/2-inch (13 mm) needle or 31 G 13 mm.

- Pressure regulator
- Carboxytherapy device
- Particle filter
- Connection tubes
- 30–31G needles

Follow the required intradermal/subdermal sterile technique.

TECHNIQUE

First of all, there has to be a full clinical evaluation, diagnosis, a detailed assessment of the skin and the aesthetics that has to be treated. The treating physician has to define the volume to be used according to the pathology and deepness to be treated. Always use warm gas (usually the machine is automatically set to 28°C, as cold air is very painful and not to be injected). Then choose the right flow, according to the area and patient's personal and local sensitivity. The environmental air of the system should always be purged, so that it contains only CO_2. If the tubing system contains ambiental air, too much inflammation may occur. Local anesthesia is advisable. The needle should be introduced with a 45° angle into the skin with a sterile technique. For intradermal treatment, the angle should be less. The needle has to be attached through the connecting tube to the carboxytherapy device. Only then, the treating physician is ready to push the button or pedal and start the injection of the gas.

Volumes to be used depend on the pathology or inaesthetics.

It is best to do treatments every 2–3 weeks depending on the diagnosis. Most patients will get skin improvements after 2–3 weeks of treatment. When treating subdermal fat, best results are obtained in 10 weeks **(Fig. 2)**.

ADVANTAGES

The treatment should be done by a trained physician, not by a nonmedical professional. Furthermore, this procedure cannot be performed in a

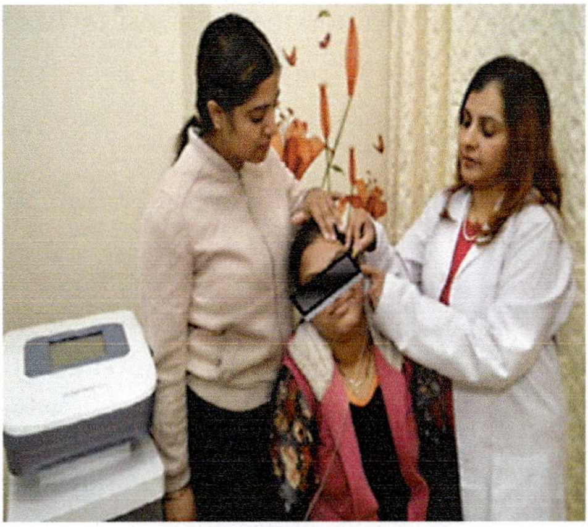

Fig. 2: Carboxytherapy for under eye circles.
Source: Jindal P. et al.; 2020 (with permission)

nonmedical facility. It is a minimal invasive treatment, completely outpatient with fast sessions (not more than 20 minutes) and small areas can be treated without anesthesia. If done properly, there should be no side effects. One of the greatest advantages is that residual adiposities, such those left after a liposuction, can be treated and the body contour can be regularized.

The periocular area is of concern because of flaccidity, wrinkles, and dark circles. Carboxytherapy is a very good tool to treat these issues.

Carboxytherapy devices are inexpensive and require little maintenance. CO_2 is also an inexpensive gas. It is very important to invest in good machine.

DISADVANTAGES

First of all, many sessions are required. Some patients may feel impatient. It is important to set real expectations on the clinical results of this minimal invasive treatment. Treating patients with very high expectations is not recommended.

Few patients dislike some of the side effects, like swelling under eye for 1–2 days due to accumulated CO_2 even though they are mild, transient and well tolerated by the great majority of patients.

Most of the devices do not require maintenance, but for some automatic devices technical support is needed.

SIDE EFFECTS

Side effects are mild, transient and well tolerated by the vast majority of patients:

- Crackling sensation in the area of injection that lasts for 1–2 hours
- Pain at the site of injection (about 75% of the patients); it is handled by heating the gas up to 28°C and decreasing the flow

- Hematomas at the site of injection that may last up to 4 days and are not of aesthetic concern

AESTHETIC INDICATIONS

Carboxytherapy is widely used in aesthetic medicine to treat various skin and body concerns, including:

- *Cellulite reduction:* Carboxytherapy is used among other treatments, because its unique effect on the subdermal adipose layer.[8,10,11] Its infusion into the affected site produces mesolipolysis and aims to remove cellulite and improve skin texture.[9] Carboxytherapy is effective to treat buttocks, thighs, abdomen and local adiposities of the knees[6,9,10]
  By improving microcirculation and lymphatic drainage, carboxytherapy helpsreduce the appearance of cellulite.
- *Localized fat deposits:* It affects young and old patients; and residual adiposities may remain after a liposuction surgical procedure.[12] Carboxytherapy is an excellent tool for body contouring.

  Carboxytherapy produces a lipoclastic effect on fat tissue, as demonstrated without effects on the blood vessels or nerves and it is a secure procedure.[13] A 30-G needle is best for this treatment, since higher flow can be used in this area (up to 200 cc/min) and higher volumes are required as well; depending on the size of the adiposity 200–1,000 cc. Remember to never use more than 2 L in one session, since the patient may get dizzy due to transient hypercapnia. It is often used in conjunction with other treatments to target small areas of fat accumulation, such as under the chin or around the abdomen.
- *Stretch marks:* Stretch marks (striae distensae) are fractures of collagen fibers within the dermis (dermal scars). It showed thickening and an increase and rearrangement of collagen fibers in the dermis after CO_2 treatment[1,12] and Hodeib[16] showed an increase of fibronectin in stretch marks.[14,15] Carboxytherapy promotes collagen production, which can improve the texture and appearance of stretch marks.
- *Dark circles:* By increasing circulation and oxygenation around the eyes, carboxytherapy helps reduce the appearance of dark circles.
- *Skin rejuvenation:* Because its effect on dermal collagen, CO_2 may be used in any area of the body.[7] With multiple punctures and low CO_2 doses separated by a few centimeters.[6] The procedure is commonly used for antiaging purposes, as it stimulates collagen and improves skin elasticity, reducing wrinkles and sagging.

MEDICAL INDICATIONS

Beyond aesthetics, carboxytherapy has therapeutic applications in the treatment of several medical conditions. Initially developed to improve blood flow in patients with vascular conditions, carboxytherapy is still used in this context. The treatment accelerates wound healing by enhancing tissue oxygenation and nutrient delivery in chronic wounds. Carboxytherapy may be beneficial in the treatment of skin disorders such as psoriasis, where improved blood flow and skin regeneration are helpful. It promotes healing and regeneration of tissues, making it useful for treating scars and ulcers, particularly when other treatments have failed.

CONCLUSION

Carboxytherapy is a versatile, minimally invasive treatment that has demonstrated efficacy in both aesthetic and medical applications. It offers a safe and effective alternative to more invasive procedures for conditions such as cellulite, localized fat, stretch marks, and skin laxity. However, it is not without limitations, including the need for multiple sessions and the potential for mild side effects. Proper patient selection, adherence to technique, and awareness of contraindications are crucial for achieving the best results.

REFERENCES

1. Jindal P, Malhotra N, Joshi S (Eds.). Aesthetic and Regenerative Gynecology, Springer Publication; 2022. [online] Available from https://doi.org/10.1007/978-981-16-1743-0_11[Last accessed December, 2024].
2. Yoshitada S, Miwa M, Oe K, Ueha T, Koh A, Niikura T, et al. A novel system for transcutaneous application of carbon dioxide causing an "artificial Bohr effect" in the human body. PLoS One. 2011;6(9):e24137.
3. D'Arcangelo D, Facchiano F, Barlucchi LM, Melillo G, Illi B, Testolin L, et al. Acidosis inhibits endothelial cell apoptosis and function and induces basic fibroblast growth factor and vascular endothelial growth factor expression. Circ Res. 2000;86(3):312-8.
4. Brandi C, D'Aniello C, Grimaldi L, Bosi B, Dei I, Lattarulo P, et al. Carbon dioxide therapy in the treatment of localized adiposities: clinical study and hystopathological correlations. Aesthetic Plast Surg. 2001;25:170-4.
5. Bunyatyan ND, Drogovoz SM, Kononenko AV, Prokofiev AB. Carboxytherapy - An Innovative Trend in Resort Medicine. Vopr Kurortol Fizioter Lech Fiz Kult. 2018;95(5):72-6.
6. Kołodziejczak A, Podgórna K, Rotsztejn H. Is carboxytherapy a good alternative method in the removal of various skin defects? Dermatol Ther. 2018;31(5):e12699.
7. Koutná N. Carboxytherapy in Aesthetic Medicine. Aesthetic Med; 2011.pp. 547-76.
8. Ordiz I. Técnicas combinadas empleadas en el Rejuvenecimiento Facial. Oviedo; 2013.pp. 106-8.
9. Draelos ZD, Marenus KD. Cellulite. Etiology and purported treatment. Dermatol Surg. 1997;23:1177-81.
10. Eldsouky F, Ebrahim HM. Evaluation and efficacy of carbon dioxide therapy (carboxytherapy) versus mesolipolysis in the treatment of cellulite. J Cosmet Laser Ther. 2018;20(5):307-12.

11. Atamoros FMP, Pérez DA, Sigall DA, Romay AAA, Gastelum JAB, de la Peña Salcedo JA , et al. Evidence-based treatment for gynoid lipodystrophy: A review of the recent literature. J Cosmet Dermatol. 2018;17(6):977-83.
12. Balik O, Yilmaz M, Bagriyanik A. Does carbon dioxide therapy really diminish localized adiposities? Experimental study with rats. Aesthetic Plast Surg. 2011;35:470-4.
13. Brandi C, D'Aniello C. Carbon dioxide therapy: effects on skin irregularity and its use a complement to liposuction, Aesthetic Plast Surg. 2004;28:222-5.
14. Brandi C, Grimaldi L, Nisi G, Brafa A, Campa A, Calabrò M, et al. The role of carbon dioxide therapy in the treatment of chronic wounds. In Vivo. 2010;24(2):223-6.
15. Brandi C, Campana M, Russo F, Brafa A, Nisi G, Grimaldi L, et al. Carbon dioxide: maybe not the only one but an efficient and secure gas for treating local adiposities. Aesthetic Plast Surg. 2012;36:218-9.
16. Hodeib AA, Hassan GFR, Ragab MNM, Hasby EA. Clinical and immunohistochemical comparative study of the efficacy of carboxytherapy vs platelet-rich plasma in treatment of stretch marks. J Cosmet Dermatol. 2018;17(6):1008-15.

13

CHAPTER

Platelet-rich Plasma Therapy: A Perspective into Treating Gynecological Disorders

Prabhu Chandra Mishra, Neharika Malhotra

HISTORY OF PLATELET-RICH PLASMA

The use of platelet-rich plasma (PRP) which is described as plasma with higher platelet count than that of peripheral blood dates back to 1970s when hematologists used it to treat thrombocytopenia. PRP is also commonly termed as PRF (Platelet-rich fibrin) matrix, GF-s (Platelet-rich growth factors), and platelet concentrate.[1,2] Over the years, the field has witnessed the use of PRP widely for tissue regeneration, skin rejuvenation, scars and wound healing, and for alopecia treatment owing to its property to kick start healing cascade.[3-8]

The success of PRP in maxillofacial surgery as PRF, a decade later, was due to the potential of fibrin for adherence and homeostatic properties, and of PRP to stimulate cell proliferation.[9] Subsequent studies had shown remarkable recovery and complete pain relief when PRP injections were given for athletic injuries.[10] Hence, the use of PRP therapy for the treatment of musculoskeletal diseases such as arthritis, tendonitis, tears, and ligament sprains was promoted, thereby, making PRP therapy highly prevalent in orthopedic and sports medicine.[11]

Histological evidence suggested that when PRP is injected in deep dermis and immediate subdermis, it induces activation of fibroblasts, soft-tissue augmentation, new collagen deposition, adipose tissue formation, and formation of new blood vessels. This led PRP therapy to become a popular and reliable procedure in cosmetic dermatology field.[12,13] With the remarkable success of PRP due to its natural healing properties, other medical fields that use PRP are gynecology, pediatric surgery, cardiac surgery, ophthalmology, plastic surgery, and urology.[14,15]

UNDERSTANDING PLATELET-RICH PLASMA

Platelets are tiny blood cells called thrombocytes which are made in bone marrow. Initially, the only property attributed to platelets was to maintain homeostasis, however, with time, the research has shown that these cells have a plethora of functions and the abilities to their name. Platelets are known to be rich in cytokines, coagulation factors, adhesion molecules, immunologic molecules, and regulators of growth and angiogenesis which have peculiar roles in inflammatory processes, coagulation and immunity modulation. They promote angiogenesis, tissue remodeling, and aid in wound healing process.[16] It is due to these aspects, that PRP represents a novel therapeutic option for the treatment of a large number of diseases.

Platelet Biology

The initiation of repair and regenerative process inside the body is marked by the formation of a blood clot which is facilitated by the platelets also called thrombocytes. These are the smallest in size in comparison to other cell types found in the blood and have no nucleus. The main function of platelets in the cell is maintaining homeostasis by adhesion and aggregation leading to the formation of primary platelet plug. Additionally, platelets synthesize, store, and release various compounds such as: thrombin, serotonin, adenine nucleotides, Ca^{2+} ions. They aid in vascular wall remediation, triggering of inflammatory response, immune response, and wound healing partly by acting as a reservoir of a vast number of growth factors **(Fig. 1)**.

The key growth factors stored in platelets are:

- *Platelet-derived growth factor (PDGF):* It was originally discovered as the main constituent of platelets. Although α-granules of platelets are the

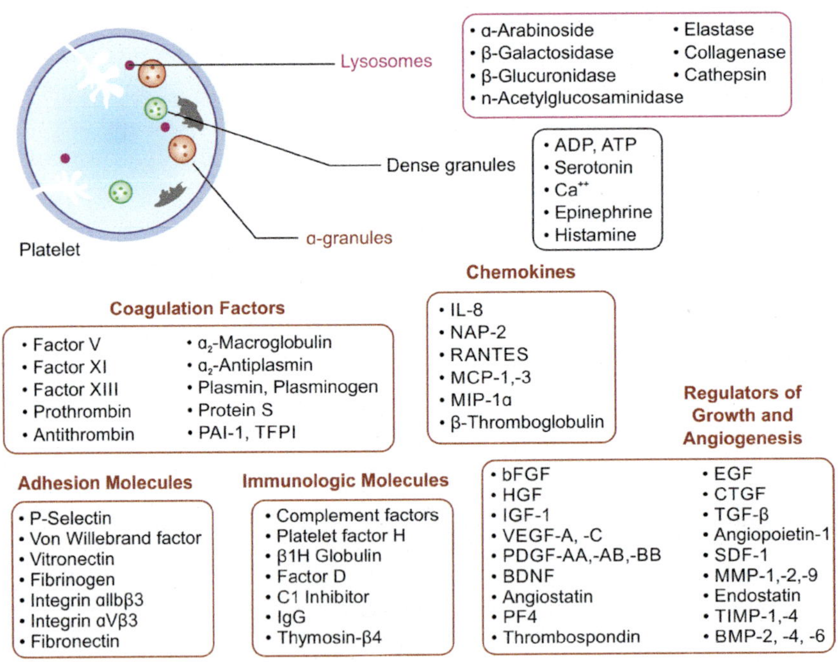

Fig. 1: Platelet composition (needs to be remade).

main storage site for PDGF, it is also produced by other cell types such as fibroblasts, endothelial cells, keratinocytes, and macrophages. PDGF stimulates cell growth, affects chemotaxis and differentiation of specific cell types while promoting cell survival. The chemotactic effect of platelets cannot only be observed on the stem cells present in the bone marrow but also on fibroblasts, monocytes, and neutrophils. PDGF activates fibroblasts for proliferation and for the production of components of extracellular matrix. Direct application of PDGF for wound healing causes rapid healing of the wound, leads to the appearance of granulation tissue, and also increases mechanical strength of the skin. Studies have shown a reduction of PDGF levels in cases of delayed healing and diabetic foot. Due to the effects of platelets, it has vital role in stimulation of wound healing cascade, maintenance of connective tissue homeostasis, and in certain organs during embryonic development.

- *Transforming growth factor β (TGF-β):* It is produced mainly by the platelets just after tissue injury and is involved in wound healing and scarring. It has three known isoforms and is a vital player in cell proliferation, differentiation, and apoptosis. In endothelial cells, TGF-β is activated by retinoic acid and FGF-2 (Fibroblast growth factor-2) and in macrophages by endotoxin and bleomycin. Moreover, a variety of molecules are involved in its activation. This cytokine plays a role in synthesis stimulation and degradation of extracellular matrix proteins. It further regulates cells' entry into the apoptosis pathway.
- *Epidermal growth factor (EGF):* EGF is present in the α-granules of human platelets. Its stimulates the migration and proliferation of epidermal cells. Its function is to accelerate skin metabolism and promotes the transport of active nutrients, resulting in increased collagen synthesis. Moreover, it is also responsible for repairing damaged polysaccharides and glycoproteins that build cell membranes.[8]
- *Fibroblast growth factor (FGF):* Active mitogen, which stimulates the proliferation of many cells. Basic fibroblast growth factor (FGF-2) is an especially important factor—it is produced by damaged endothelial cells of the blood vessels immediately after injury or severe burns. It stimulates mature endothelial cells and their precursors to migration and mitotic division.[9]
- *Vascular endothelial growth factor (VEGF):* One of the most active angiogenesis and vasculogenesis inducers, in addition to thrombocytes produced in keratinocytes, macrophages, fibroblasts and neutrophils. This cytokine acts via receptors mainly on the surface of endothelial cells, triggering the signal that stimulates angiogenesis. This results in the construction of new vessels on the scaffold composed of collagen and other proteins of the extracellular matrix. VEGF was also shown

to participate in the production of collagen fibers and stimulation of thrombocyte agglomeration and clot formation.

- *Insulin-like growth factor (IGF):* Its activity mainly involves the activation of keratinocytes and the stimulation of epidermal cell proliferation.
- *Hepatocyte growth factor (HGF):* Responsible for regulating migration and differentiating stem cells of the epidermis. Due to the particularly high content of these factors in the formulations of PRP, they have been used in various fields of medicine, including the treatment of chronic, difficult to heal wounds, soft tissue injuries, maxillofacial surgery, implantology, periodontics, burns, plastic surgery and aesthetic dermatology as one of the main antiaging therapies.

Studies have shown that growth factors are present in significantly higher amounts in PRP as compared to platelet poor plasma and whole blood. PRP has been shown to promote changes in monocyte-mediated proinflammatory chemokine/cytokine release.[17] The levels of Lipoxin A4 (LXA4) are also found to be significantly higher in PRP compared to whole blood. LXA4 is an endogenous lipoxygenase-derived eicosanoid mediator that has been shown to possess dual pro-resolving and anti-inflammatory properties. According to the study, PRP suppresses the cytokine release, limits inflammation and henceforth promotes tissue regeneration.[17]

Platelet growth factors are responsible for only a part of platelet bioactivity. Along with the growth factors and other signaling molecules, platelets function with red blood cells and leukocytes to ignite the repair process, and the duration and magnitude of the inflammatory response is dictated by their cooperative engagement.

PRP FOR THE TREATMENT OF THIN ENDOMETRIUM AND OVARIAN REJUVENATION

Premature ovarian failure (POF) is one of the leading causes of premature menopause and is diagnosed in approximately 1% women aged under 40 years. The onset of premature menopause is also attributed several other factors such as family history, behavioral habits like smoking, chemotherapy or pelvic radiation treatments for cancer, autoimmune diseases, chronic fatigue syndrome, etc.[18] Women who experience premature menopause are at a higher risk of neurological diseases, psychosexual dysfunction, osteoporosis, mood disorders, ischemic heart disease, infertility and premature death.[19] The treatments that are readily available at hand to mitigate some of these adverse outcomes include estrogen treatment which can be initiated after the onset of menopause or hormone replacement therapy.

In scenarios where patients with irregular menstrual cycles or showing the symptoms of menstruation absence wish to address the concern of infertility, may consider the option of oocyte cryopreservation to preserve their fertility or in vitro fertilization (IVF) treatment but the success of these treatments in the light of premature menopause onset is almost impossible to achieve. In such cases, the patients turn to oocyte donation or adoption as their only options available. Such kind of alternative options may not be welcomed by some patients based on their personal values and desire.[20]

Another cause for infertility could be premature ovarian insufficiency (POI) which occurs before a woman turns 40 years of age. The women witness elevated levels of serum follicle-stimulating hormone (FSH) (FSH >40 IU/L) and an associated cessation of menstruation. In addition, profound hypoestrogenism is observed which has detrimental effects in the body.[21] Patients with POI face the challenge of reproducing using their own gametes and oocyte donation has been the only recommended and proven treatment for women with POI. Taking the defined course of these treatments, it is still difficult to predict pregnancy outcome post-assisted reproductive technology (ART). The other parameters which affect the outcome are maternal age, ovarian reserve measurement and endometrial receptivity (ER). ER is evaluated with a traditional two-dimensional (2D) ultrasound which assesses endometrial thickness (Eth) and endometrial pattern (EnP). Eth of <7 mm on ultrasound is considered as a thin endometrium which usually results in cycle cancellation and hence is nonresponsive to standard treatments posing a challenge in ART.[22] Numerous strategies have been utilized for the treatment of thin endometrium such as use of low-dose aspirin, use of exogenous estrogen, vitamin E, electroacupuncture, vaginal sildenafil citrate, and application of granulocyte colony-stimulation factor (G-CSF). Ironically despite performing these remedies, many women do not respond to the ART.[23-25]

PRP in Treating Thin Endometrium

The successful use of PRP in improving endometrium thickness in the patients undergoing IVF treatment was first reported in 2015 by Chang et al.[26] According to the study, after standard hormone replacement therapy, five patients still had to cancel embryo transfer cycle due to poor endometrial response (Eth <7 mm). The group performed intrauterine infusion of PRP post which endometrial expansion was observed. Embryos were transferred and successful pregnancy was observed in all the patients.[26] Another study performed by Zadehmodarres et al.[27] reported the effectiveness of PRP for endometrial growth in patients with a thin endometrium. This group performed the study with 10 patients with a history of cancelled cycles because of inadequate endometrial growth (Eth < 7 mm). They found that at 48 hours post first PRP application, endometrial thickness increased which reached more than 7 mm after the second PRP application in all the patients. Five patients became pregnant (50%) after frozen embryo transfer (FET), and in four of them the pregnancy progressed normally.[27]

Kim et al. (2019)[28] conducted a pilot study to unravel the effect of PRP therapy on thin endometrium. They considered women who presented with a history of failed IVF cycles atleast twice, refractory thin endometrium [endometrial thickness (EMT) <7 mm], undergone more than two cycles of previous therapy for increasing the EMT, such as, hysteroscopic adhesiolysis following hormone replacement therapy, high dose estradiol valerate, transvaginal sildenafil administration, or pentoxifylline combination with vitamin E, and frozen embryo available for embryo transfer. Intrauterine autologous PRP administration was performed at the estrogen-primed FET cycle. The first autologous PRP infusion was performed on menstrual cycle day 10 which was repeated at 3 days intervals until the thickness of endometrium reached 7 mm. ET was conducted 3 days after the final autologous PRP administration. The serum β-hCG levels were measured from peripheral blood 2 weeks after ET. The authors found that the use of autologous PRP significantly improved implantation, pregnancy, and live birth rates of the patients with refractory thin endometrium.[28]

Furthermore, a study conducted using an animal model by Jang et al.,[29] investigated the role of PRP in the endometrium regeneration after ethanol-induced damage. They observed that intrauterine administration of autologous PRP not only stimulated but it also accelerated regeneration of the endometrium which was coupled with decreasing fibrosis in a murine model of endometrial damage.[29]

PRP in Ovarian Rejuvenation

Platelet-rich plasma therapy is an emerging promising treatment in the reproductive context as it enhances the development of primordial and primary preantral follicles.[30] PRP has not only been proven to prevent possible ischemia following ovarian injury, but it is explicitly clear that the use of PRP to target various issues regarding the reproductive system is highly positive and beneficial. According to a report by Sfakianoudis et al. in 2019,[31] autologous PRP application lead to pregnancy in menopause for a woman aged 40 and diagnosed with premature menopause. The patient chose PRP therapy with the aim to rejuvenate the ovarian tissue to enable the employment of her own gametes through IVF. The results showed a significant reduction in FSH levels after 6 weeks following the autologous PRP treatment.[31]

Recently Melo et al. in 2020[32] studied the impact of intracortical injections of autologous PRP on ovarian reserve markers in women observed with low ovarian reserve before undergoing ART. A significant improvement in the levels of FSH, antral follicle count (AFC) , and anti-Müllerian hormone (AMH) was seen with no change in the control group. The group concluded that PRP injections improved these markers of low ovarian reserve, and the therapy was safe and effective.[32]

Sfakianoudis et al. in 2020[33] performed a study to investigate the impact of PRP application for ovarian rejuvenation. Four pilot studies were conducted on poor ovarian response (POR), premature ovarian insufficiency (POI), perimenopause, and menopause, respectively. Primary outcome measures for the POR pilot study were levels of AMH, AFC and oocyte yield. For the POI, perimenopausal and menopausal pilot studies primary outcome measures were restoration of menstrual cycle, and FSH levels. A significant improvement on the hormonal profile and the ovarian reserve status was noted, along with improved intracytoplasmic sperm injection (ICSI) cycle performance concerning POR participants. Menstruation recovery was observed along with a statistically significant improvement on levels of AMH, FSH, and AFC. Similarly, significant number of menopausal women positively responded to PRP treatment. Finally, menstruation regularity, improved hormonal levels and AFC were reported for perimenopausal women. The group concluded that PRP infusion shows promising results in addressing ovarian insufficiency.[33]

PREPARATION OF PLATELET-RICH PLASMA

There is no consensus regarding PRP preparation. PRP is prepared through a process known as differential centrifugation, which separated the components of blood based on different specific gravity.[34] The preparation of PRP depends on the type of device chosen and should be done according to the manufacturer's instructions. There are different PRP systems that facilitate the preparation of PRP in a reproducible manner. All operate on a small volume of drawn blood and on the principle of centrifugation **(Table 1)**.

Even though most devices aim to obtain the best PRP, the systems differ widely in their ability to collect and concentrate platelets depending on the methodology, speed and time of centrifugation. Consequently, suspensions of different concentrations of platelets and leukocytes are obtained.[34]

Methodology

We follow our own protocol for PRP preparation for conducting our studies which is as follows:

- Venous blood (15–50 mL) is drawn from the patient's arm in anti-coagulant-containing tubes
- The recommended temperature during processing is 21–24°C to prevent platelet activation during centrifugation of the blood
- The blood is centrifuged at 1,800 rpm for 12 minutes
- The blood separates into three layers: an upper layer that contains platelets and white blood cells, an intermediate thin layer (the buffy coat) that is rich in white blood cells, and a bottom layer that contains red blood cells **(Fig. 2)**

TABLE 1: Devices and coagulant used.

Devices	*Blood collection/ anticoagulant*	*Centrifugation*		
		Number of times	*Speed/time*	*Centrifuge*
Selphyl®	Tube 9 mL/sodium citrate	1	1,100 g/6 minutes	Classic
PRGF Endoret®	Tube 9 mL/sodium citrate	1	270 g/7 minutes	Classic
Cascade®	Tube 9 mL/sodium citrate	2	1,100 g/6 minutes 1,450 g/15 minutes	Classic
Plateltex®	Tube 9 mL/ACD	2	180 g/10 minutes 1,000 g/10 minutes	Classic
Regenkit®	Tube 9 mL/sodium citrate	1	1,500 g/9 minutes	Classic
ACP Arthrex®	Syringe 15 mL/ACD or no anticoagulant	1	1,500 rpm/5 minutes	Adapted
GPS III®	Syringe 30 or 60 mL/ ACD	1	3,200 rpm/15 minutes	Adapted
Genesis®	Syringe 12 mL/ACD	1	2,400 rpm/12 minutes	Adapted
SmartPrep 2®	Syringe 20 or 60 mL/ ACD	2	2,500 rpm/4 minutes 2,300 rpm/10 minutes	Adapted
Proteal®	Syringe 20 mL/ sodium citrate	1	1,800 rpm/8 minutes	Adapted
Magellan®	Syringe 30–60 mL/ ACD	–	–	Adapted device
Angel®	Syringe 40–180 mL/ ACD	–	–	Adapted device

(ACD: acid citrate dextrose).
Courtesy: Dr Jeremy Magalon, adapted from Dohan Ehrenfest

- The upper and intermediate buffy layers are transferred to an empty sterile tube. The plasma is centrifuged again at 3,200 rpm for 6 minutes to help with the formation of soft pellets (erythrocytes and platelets) at the bottom of the tube
- The upper two-thirds of the plasma is discarded because it is platelet-poor plasma
- Pellets are homogenized in the lower third (5 mL) of the plasma to create the PRP
- The PRP is now ready for injection. Approximately 30 mL of venous blood yields 3–5 mL of PRP

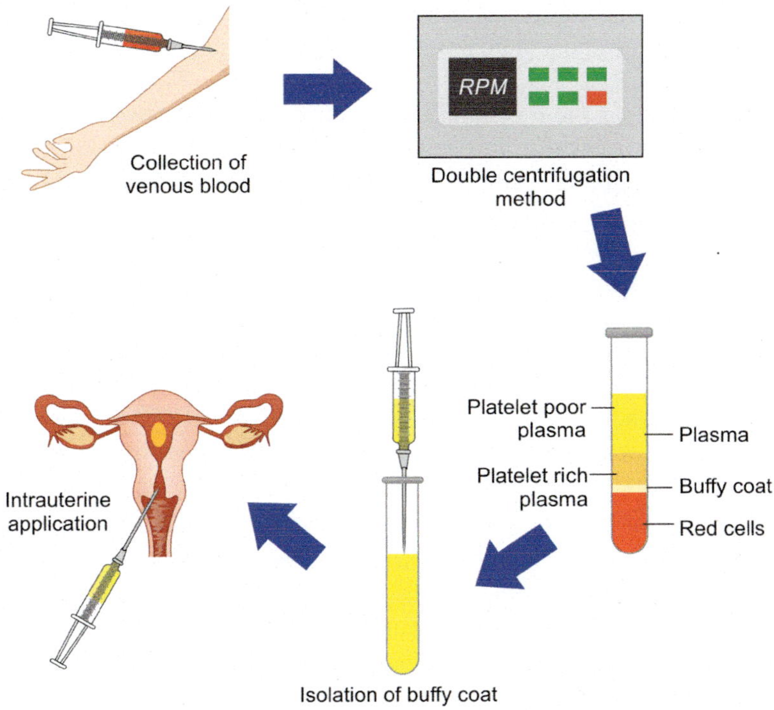

Fig. 2: *Schematic representation of the protocol for platelet-rich plasma (PRP) preparation and collection for application.* Venous blood is collected and subjected to double centrifugation method to separate the components of the blood. After centrifugation, the blood components (red blood cells, leukocytes, and platelets) are separated from the plasma due to their different densities. The platelets have the lowest density and hence float on top. The yellow part consisting of PRP is then collected via syringes and to heal premenopausal issues, is subjected to intrauterine application.

- We then inject the prepared PRP either laparoscopically (2.5 cc in each ovary) at multiple site but preferably at cortex stromal site and sometimes in medulla of ovary in case of ovarian atrophy.

PLATELET-RICH PLASMA COMPOSITION AND ACTIVATION

Since PRP has high level of platelets, it is abundant in chemokines, growth factors, cytokines, plasma proteins which are stored within α-granules and other biomolecules such as fibronectin, vitronectin, and sphingosine 1-phosphate. The growth factors include insulin-like growth factor, platelet-derived growth factor, platelet-derived angiogenic factor, vascular endothelial growth factor, fibroblast growth factor, transforming growth factor beta, connective tissue growth factor, epidermal growth factor, and interleukin-8.

Altogether, the vast variety of active signaling molecules found in PRP is responsible for the onset of inflammation, stem cell migration, angiogenesis, and cell proliferation.[3,35,37]

Platelet-rich plasma is composed of neutrophils, monocyte macrophages which are highly motile and migrate to the site, fibroblasts: produce collagen, glycosaminoglycans, reticular fibers, and glycoprotein; endothelial cells which act as permeability barrier, regulate vascular reactivity, vasoconstrictors, vasodilators, inflammation, and immunity; keratinocytes whose main function is to act as barrier; hematopoietic stem cells (HSCs) which are multipotent in nature.[36,38]

Platelet-rich plasma activation can be done exogenously with the use of thrombin, calcium chloride, and collagen or through mechanical trauma. Each method of activation influences the physical form of PRP, bioavailability of PRP, the amount of growth factors released, and the kinetics of release.[39]

PROPOSED MECHANISM OF ACTION

With the success of PRP therapy in treating many diseases as documented in **Table 2** in addition to gynecological disorders, elucidating the molecular mechanism of action of PRP is crucial. According to the recent study, formation of regenerative matrix is supported by the fibrin framework present over platelets.[40] It is known that higher concentration of growth factors in PRP promote the initiation of the healing cascade.[38] The ignition of the process starting from tissue necrosis resolution, chemotaxis, cell regeneration, cell proliferation and migration to extracellular matrix synthesis, remodeling, angiogenesis, and epithelialization is attributed to the release of various growth factors such as TGF-β, PDGF, IGF, VEGF, EGF and FGF-2, and differentiation factors like GDF-9 (growth differentiation factor 9) upon platelet activation **(Figs. 3A and B).** GDF-9 serves as a biomarker for oocyte maturation and its mutations have been linked to premature ovarian failure.[41-43]

Ovary is highly angiogenic in structure and platelet-derived factors play a crucial role in vascular activation and stabilization. The proposed mechanism of PRP application to treat ovarian insufficiency, premature menopause or thin endometrium, may involve the enrichment of the ovarian tissue with essential factors required for neoangiogenesis. Moreover, as shown in the studies Virant-Klun et al. 2008,[44] very small embryonic-like stem cells (VSELs) and ovarian stem cells (OSCs) or germline stem cells (GSCs) are detected in human ovarian surface epithelium even in the case of postmenopausal and premature ovarian failure women. Surprisingly, these stem cells/germline stem cells retain the ability to differentiate into oocytes under certain conditions which paves a new direction for the origin of PRP-derived follicles.[44]

TABLE 2: Evidence-based studies related to the application of platelet-rich plasma (PRP).

Application	*Evidence-based studies*
PRP in skin lesion and wound healing	PRP to promote angiogenesis and wound healing and it was tested by Tehranian et al.[45] in wound healing in high-risk women undergoing cesarean sections. They applied PRP in 70 patients and compared them to 71 control cases without PRP application. They found a greater reduction in the redness, edema, ecchymosis, discharge, approximation score than in the control group
PRP in cervical ectopy	Hua et al.[46] conducted a randomized clinical study to compare the effectiveness of autologous PRP application to that of laser treatment for benign cervical ectopy. They applied PRP twice on the area of cervical erosion with a 1-week interval in 60 patients, while laser treatment was used in the other 60 patients. They found that the complete cure rate was 93.7% in the PRP group and the mean time to re-epithelialization was significantly shorter in the PRP and the rate of adverse treatment effects was much lower in the PRP group than in the laser group
PRP in O-shot therapy	Neto JB et al.[47] conducted a study to evaluate the safety, tolerability and clinical efficacy of "O-Shot" PRP of the vulvovaginal field among 68 women with symptoms of stress incontinence (13 patients), overactive bladder (15 patients), mixed (22 patients), lack of lubrication and sexual dysfunction (libido, arousal, dyspareunia). Treatment protocol was based on two sessions of PRP (O-Shot) two months apart. The study concluded that PRP, "O-Shot" is an in-office treatment that is safe, effective, non-surgical, and nonhormonal option for women having stress incontinence, overactive bladder, lack of lubrication, and sexual dysfunction, such as lack of libido, arousal or dyspareunia
PRP in vaginal rejuvenation	Kim et al.[48] reported the use of PRP in a case of vaginal rejuvenation. They concluded that the application of autologous lipofilling mixed with PRP in a patient with vaginal atrophy produced relief of symptoms and contour restoration. The rejuvenated appearance of the external genitalia provided a pleasing cosmetic outcome to the patient
PRP in vulvar lichen sclerosis	Goldstein et al.[49] showed that among 15 patients with biopsy proven vulvar lichen sclerosus (VLS) received two separate treatments of PRP separated by 6 weeks. It was observed that out of 12 patients, 7 had decreased inflammation on their post-treatment biopsies which statistically significant

Contd...

Contd…

Application	*Evidence-based studies*
PRP in breast reconstruction	Gentile et al.[50] enrolled 100 patients aged between 19 and 60 years affected by breast soft-tissue defects. They divided the patients into two equally-sized groups. The study group was treated with fat grafting and PRP, while the control group was treated with fat grafting injections only. They found that the patients treated with PRP added to the autologous fat grafts showed a 69% maintenance rate of the restored contour and of three-dimensional volume after 1 year. They concluded that PRP mixed with fat grafts led to improvements in the maintenance of breast volume in patients affected by breast soft-tissue defects. Similar results were obtained by Salgarello et al[51]
PRP in premature ovarian failure	PRP therapy is investigated in women with POF, infertile women more than 35 years of age, and women with low ovarian reserve. PRP is injected into the ovary under ultrasound guidance, Pantos et al.[52] at the annual European Society of Human Reproduction and Embryology conference held in 2016 in Helsinki, Finland, introduced this modality (ovarian rejuvenation). They injected PRP in eight perimenopausal/POF women with poor ovarian reserve. They found successful ovarian rejuvenation 1–3 months after PRP treatment. All cases underwent natural IVF cycles with follicles of 15.20 ± 2.05 mm in diameter, the resulting oocytes were inseminated by intracytoplasmic sperm injection (ICSI), and all resulting embryos were cryopreserved
PRP in refractory endometrium	Colombo et al.[53] and Zadehmodarres et al.[27] in their respective studies, showed that endometrial thickness increased at 48 hours after the first PRP application and reached more than 7 mm after the second PRP application in all patients. They concluded that PRP was effective for endometrial growth in patients with a refractory endometrium
PRP in genital fistulae	Adler et al.[54] in his systemic review, that assessed conservative and surgical treatments found that small fistulae could be treated conservatively with various therapies, including PRP, with success rates ranging from 67 to 100%. Shirvan et al.[55] concluded that autologous PRP injection and PRF glue interposition offered a safe, effective, and novel minimally invasive approach for the treatment of vesicovaginal fistulae that obviated the need for open surgery
PRP in genital prolapse and urinary incontinence	PRP mixture causes rapid remodeling and connective tissue growth after vaginal surgery and because of this property Gorlero et al.[56] in his observational study of 10 consecutive women requiring surgery for prolapse recurrence were operated on the cases and performed PRF injections. The success rate was 80% with complete symptom relief. Sexual activity increased by 20% without dyspareunia. They concluded that the use of PRF for site-specific prolapse repair was associated with good functional outcomes

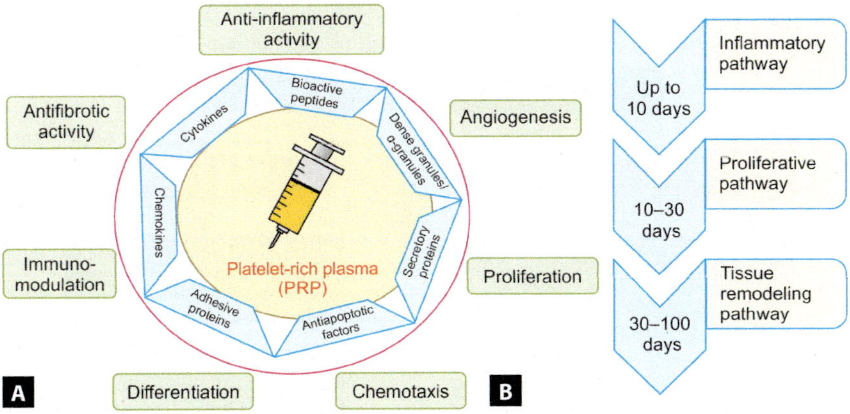

Figs. 3A and B: *Mechanism of action of platelet-rich plasma* (PRP). (A) The figure depicts the composition of PRP and the various pathways that it is predicted to target to initiate the healing cascade; (B) The timeline of the PRP-induced process. The flowchart signifies when to repeat the next cycle of PRP.

APPLICATIONS OF PLATELET-RICH PLASMA

Platelet-rich plasma application has seen the light of success not only in ovarian rejuvenation and in treating premature menopausal conditions, but also it is applied for many other conditions as shown in **Flowchart 1**.

Furthermore, **Table 2** provides the evidence-based studies where PRP related to applications of PRP.

CONTRAINDICATIONS AND ADVERSE EFFECTS

- Individuals who smoke
- Individuals who have skin cancer
- Individuals who have liver disorders
- Individuals who have problems with blood clotting.

Adverse effects: It has been reported that PRP does not cause detectable adverse effects. There are minimal side effects or complications from PRP treatments. However, one may experience swelling, redness, and in rare cases mild bruising.[57]

FUTURE PERSPECTIVE

The future of medicine lies in harnessing the body's own potential of healing and regeneration. The advancing technologies in the field like stem cells therapy and cell-based therapy are all centered around exploiting the body's natural capacity to fight against a disease and offer treatment. PRP application in such a scenario offers a promising direction and strategy to open new avenues for treatment of a vast majority of diseases. However, the

Flowchart 1: *Applications of platelet-rich plasma (PRP).* Various therapeutic and aesthetic applications of PRP and the conditions it is used to treat under each of the areas.[10]

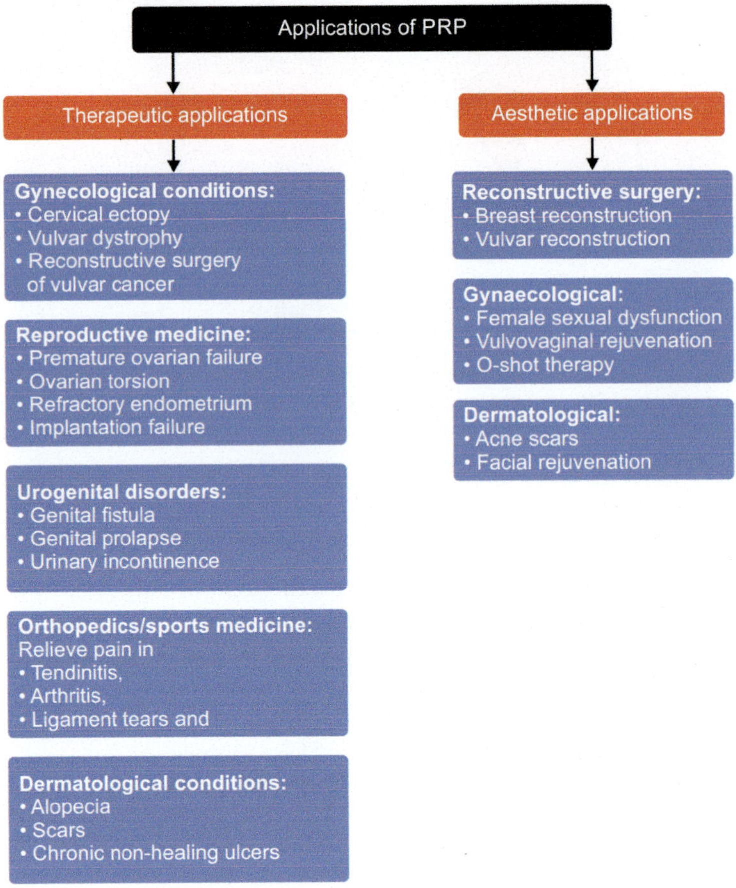

prevailing concern today is the lack of a standard uniform procedure for PRP isolation and based on the procedure followed, PRP preparation from the peripheral blood has been classified into many categories like leukocyte-rich/poor and fibrin-rich/poor. Hence, there is a need to develop protocols which can either be indication specific or a standard protocol which can be personalized based on the indication for which treatment is sought. We have developed a standard procedure for PRP preparation, and it is called O-Cell® procedure. It yields an autologous concentrate of plasma which is primarily rich in α-granules and dense granules. It is prepared by using differential centrifugation followed by double centrifugation method. The PRP preparation obtained through this procedure has enhanced regenerative and neoangiogenesis capacity.

CONCLUSION

The effectiveness of PRP is based on its high level of growth factors which are important in modulating mesenchymal cell proliferation, and extracellular matrix synthesis during the process of healing. PRP has shown to be effective at propagating new healthy tissue growth in a wide range of medical conditions.[49] During the healing process, growth factors, cytokines, and chemokines are secreted from the α-granules inside platelets. The various secreted proteins have paracrine effects on different types of cells in the body *stimulating cell migration, cell proliferation, and angiogenesis* and consequently inducing tissue regeneration.[28,58]

Platelet-rich plsma being autologous is biocompatible and nonimmunogenic in nature. It is easy to harvest, process and associated less morbidity. Low expenses are associated with its administration and therefore, PRP therapy is more affordable than other procedures. However, scientific studies done till date are only pilot studies, case reports and case series study and it necessitates for large randomized controlled studies which are required to confirm its efficacy and safety in various gynecological disorders.

REFERENCES

1. Andia I, Abate M. Platelet-rich plasma: underlying biology and clinical correlates. Regen Med. 2013;8:645-58.
2. Andia I. Platelet-rich plasma biology. In: Alves R, Grimalt R (Eds). Clinical Indications and Treatment Protocols with Platelet-Rich Plasma in Dermatology. Barcelona, Ediciones Mayo; 2016. Pp. 3-15.
3. Li ZJ, Choi HI, Choi DK, Sohn KC, Im M, Seo YJ, et al. Autologous platelet-rich plasma: a potential therapeutic tool for promoting hair growth. Dermatol Surg. 2012;38:1040-6.
4. Salazar-Álvarez AE, Riera-del-Moral LF, García-Arranz M, Alvarez-García J, Concepción-Rodriguez NA, Riera-de-Cubas L. Use of platelet-rich plasma in the healing of chronic ulcers of the lower extremity. Actas Dermosifiliogr. 2014;105:597-604.
5. Picard F, Hersant B, Bosc R, Meningaud JP. Should we use platelet-rich plasma as an adjunct therapy to treat "acute wounds", "burns", and "laser therapies": a review and a proposal of a quality criteria checklist for further studies. Wound Repair Regen. 2015;23:163-70.
6. Sclafani AP, Azzi J. Platelet preparations for use in facial rejuvenation and wound healing: a critical review of current literature. Aesthec Plast Surg. 2015;39:495-505.
7. Conde Montero E. PRP in wound healing. In: Alves R, Grimalt R (Eds). Clinical Indications and Treatment Protocols with Platelet-Rich Plasma in Dermatology. Barcelona, Ediciones Mayo; 2016. Pp. 59-72.
8. Kim DH, Je YJ, Kim CD, Lee YH, Seo YJ, Lee JH, et al. Can platelet-rich plasma be used for skin rejuvenation? Evaluation of effects of platelet-rich plasma on human dermal fibroblast. Ann Dermatol. 2011;23:424-31.
9. Conde Montero E, Fernández Santos ME, Suárez Fernández R. Platelet-rich plasma: applications in dermatology. Actas Dermosifiliogr. 2015;106:104-11.

10. Dhillon RS, Schwarz EM, Maloney MD. Platelet-rich plasma therapy: future or trend? Arthritis Res Ther. 2012;14:219.
11. Lynch MD, Bashir S. Applications of platelet-rich plasma in dermatology: a critical appraisal of the literature. J Dermatolog Treat. 2016;27:285-9.
12. Sclafani AP, McCormick SA. Induction of dermal collagenesis, angiogenesis, and adipogenesis in human skin by injection of platelet-rich fibrin matrix. Arch Facial Plast Surg. 2012;14:132-6.
13. Camps LB. PRP in cosmetic dermatology. In: Alves R, Grimalt R (Eds). Clinical Indications and Treatment Protocols with Platelet-Rich Plasma in Dermatology. Barcelona, Ediciones Mayo; 2016. Pp. 45-57.
14. Sommeling CE, Heyneman A, Hoeksema H, Verbelen J, Stillaert FB, Monstrey S. The use of platelet-rich plasma in plastic surgery: a systematic review. J Plast Reconstr Aesthet Surg. 2013;66:301-11.
15. Andia E, Rubio-Azpeitia J, Martin I, Abate M. Current concepts and translational uses of platelet rich plasma biotechnology. In: Ekinci D (Ed.). Biotechnology. In Tech; 2015.
16. Alves R, Grimalt R. A review of platelet-rich plasma: history, biology, mechanism of action, and classification. Skin Appendage Disord. 2018;4(1):18-24.
17. El-Sharkawy H, Kantarci A, Deady J, Hasturk H, Liu H, Alshahat M, et al. Platelet-rich plasma: growth factors and pro- and anti-inflammatory properties. J Periodontol. 2007;78(4):661-9.
18. Freeman EW, Sammel MD, Lin H, Gracia CR, Pien GW, Nelson DB. Symptoms associated with menopausal transition and reproductive hormones in midlife women. Obstet Gynecol. 2007;110:230-40.
19. Shuster LT, Rhodes DJ, Gostout BS, Grossardt BR, Rocca WA. Premature menopause or early menopause: Long-term health consequences. Maturitas. 2010;*65:*161-6.
20. Torrealday S, Pal L. Premature menopause. Endocrinol Metab Clin. 2015; 44:543-57.
21. Podfigurna-Stopa A, Czyzyk A, Grymowicz M, Smolarczyk R, Katulski K, Czajkowski K, et al. Premature ovarian insufficiency: the context of long-term effects. J Endocrinol Invest. 2016;39(9):983-90.
22. Mahajan N, Sharma S. The endometrium in assisted reproductive technology: How thin is thin? J Hum Reprod Sci. 2016;9(1):3.
23. Acharya S, Yasmin E, Balen AH. The use of a combination of pentoxifylline and tocopherol in women with a thin endometrium undergoing assisted conception therapies–a report of 20 cases. Hum Fertil (Camb). 2009;12:198-203.
24. Lebovitz O, Orvieto R. Treating patients with "thin" endometrium: an ongoing challenge. Gynecolendocrinol. 2014;30:409-14.
25. Zinger M, Liu JH, Thomas MA. Successful use of vaginal sildenafil citrate in two infertility patients with Asherman's syndrome. J Women's Health. 2006;15:442-4.
26. Chang Y, Li J, Chen Y, Wei L, Yang X, Shi Y, et al. Autologous platelet-rich plasma promotes endometrial growth and improves pregnancy outcome during in vitro fertilization. Int J Clin Exp Med. 2015;8(1):1286.
27. Zadehmodarres S, Salehpour S, Saharkhiz N, Nazari L. Treatment of thin endometrium with autologous platelet-rich plasma: a pilot study. JBRA Assist Reprod. 2017;21(1):54.

28. Kim H, Shin JE, Koo HS, Kwon H, Choi DH, Kim JH. Effect of autologous platelet-rich plasma treatment on refractory thin endometrium during the frozen embryo transfer cycle: a pilot study. Front Endocrinol (Lausanne). 2019;10:61.
29. Jang HY, Myoung SM, Choe JM, Kim T, Cheon YP, Kim YM, et al. Effects of autologous platelet-rich plasma on regeneration of damaged endometrium in female rats. Yonsei Med J. 2017 1;58(6):1195.
30. Hosseini L, Shirazi A, Naderi MM, Shams-Esfandabadi N, Boroujeni SB, Sarvari A, et al. Platelet-rich plasma promotes the development of isolated human primordial and primary follicles to the preantral stage. RBM Olnline. 2017;35:343-50.
31. Sfakianoudis K, Simopoulou M, Nitsos N, Rapani A, Pappas A, Pantou A, et al. Autologous platelet-rich plasma treatment enables pregnancy for a woman in premature menopause. J Clin Med. 2019;8(1):1.
32. Melo P, Navarro C, Jones C, Coward K, Coleman L. The use of autologous platelet-rich plasma (PRP) versus no intervention in women with low ovarian reserve undergoing fertility treatment: A non-randomized interventional study. J Assist Reprod Genet. 2020;7:1-9.
33. Sfakianoudis K, Simopoulou M, Grigoriadis S, Pantou A, Tsioulou P, Maziotis E, et al. Reactivating ovarian function through autologous platelet-rich plasma intraovarian infusion: pilot data on premature ovarian insufficiency, perimenopausal, menopausal, and poor responder women. J Clin Med. 2020;9(6):1809.
34. Dhurat R, Sukesh M. Principles and methods of preparation of platelet-rich plasma: a review and author's perspective. J Cutan Aesthet Surg. 2014;7:189-97.
35. Oneto P, Etulain J. PRP in wound healing applications. Platelets. 2021; 32(2):189-99.
36. Sekhon UD, Sen Gupta A. Platelets and platelet-inspired biomaterials technologies in wound healing applications. ACS Biomater Sci Eng. 2017;4(4):1176-92.
37. Textor J. Platelet-rich plasma (PRP) as a therapeutic agent: platelet biology, growth factors and a review of the literature. Platelet-rich Plasma; 2014.pp.61-94.
38. Rodrigues M, Kosaric N, Bonham CA, Gurtner GC. Wound healing: a cellular perspective. Physiol Rev. 2019;99(1):665-706.
39. Jo CH, Roh YH, Kim JE, Shin S, Yoon KS. Optimizing platelet-rich plasma gel formation by varying time and gravitational forces during centrifugation. J Oral Implantol. 2013;39:525-32.
40. Sunitha Raja V, Munirathnam Naidu E. Platelet-rich fibrin: evolution of a second-generation platelet concentrate. Indian J Dent Res. 2008;19:42-6.
41. Ferrara N, Gerber HP. The role of vascular endothelial growth factor in angiogenesis. Acta Haematol. 2001;106, 148-56.
42. Krüger JP, Freymannx U, Vetterlein S, Neumann K, Endres M, Kaps C. Bioactive factors in platelet-rich plasma obtained by apheresis. Transfus Med Hemother. 2013; 40: 432-40.
43. Otsuka F, McTavish K, Shimasaki S. Integral Role of GDF-9 and BMP-15 in Ovarian Function. Mol Reprod Dev. 2011;78:9-21.
44. Virant-Klun I, Zech N, Rožman P, Vogler A, Cvjetičanin B, Klemenc P, et al. Putative stem cells with an embryonic character isolated from the ovarian surface epithelium of women with no naturally present follicles and oocytes. Differentiation. 2008;76(8):843-56.

45. Tehranian A, Esfehani-Mehr B, Pirjani R, Rezaei N, Sadat Heidary S, Sepidarkish M. Application of autologous platelet-rich plasma (PRP) on wound healing after caesarean section in high-risk patients. Iran Red Crescent Med J. 2016;18:e34449.
46. Hua X, Zeng Y, Zhang R, Wang H, Diao J, Zhang P. Using platelet rich plasma for the treatment of symptomatic cervical ectopy. Int J Gynaecol Obstet. 2012;119:26-9.
47. Neto JB. O-Shot: Platelet rich plasma in intimate female treatment. J Womens Health Care. 2017;6:395.
48. Kim SH, Park ES, Kim TH. Rejuvenation using platelet-rich plasma and lipofilling for vaginal atrophy and lichen sclerosus. J Menopausal Med. 2017;23:63-8.
49. Goldstein AT, King M, Runels C, Gloth M, Pfau R. Intradermal injection of autologous platelet-rich plasma for the treatment of vulvar lichen sclerosus. J Am Acad Dermatol. 2017;76(1):158-60.
50. Gentile P, Di Pasquali C, Bocchini I, Floris M, Eleonora T, Fiaschetti V, et al. Breast reconstruction with autologous fat graft mixed with platelet-rich plasma. Surg Innov. 2013;20:370-6.
51. Salgarello M, Visconti G, Rusciani A. Breast fat grafting with platelet-rich plasma: a comparative clinical study and current state of the art. Plast Reconstr Surg. 2011;127:2176-85.
52. Pantos K, Nitsos N, Kokkali G, Vaxevanoglou T, Markomichali C, Pantou A, et al. Ovarian rejuvenation and folliculogenesis reactivation in peri-menopausal women after autologous platelet rich plasma treatment. Proceedings of the 32nd Annual Meeting of ESHRE. Helsinki, Finland; 2016.
53. Colombo GV, Fanton V, Sosa D, Criado Scholz E, Lotti J, Aragona SE, et al. Use of platelet rich plasma in human infertility. J Biol Regul Homeost Agents. 2017;31 (2 Suppl. 2):179-82.
54. Bodner-Adler B, Hanzal E, Pablik E, Koelbl H, Bodner K. Management of vesicovaginal fistulas (VVFs) in women following benign gynaecologic surgery: a systematic review and meta-analysis. PLoS One. 2017;12:e0171554.
55. Shirvan MK, Alamdari DH, Ghoreifi A. A novel method for iatrogenic vesicovaginal fistula treatment: autologous platelet rich plasma injection and platelet rich fibrin glue interposition. J Urol. 2013;189:2125-9.
56. Gorlero F, Glorio M, Lorenzi P, Bruno-Franco M, Mazzei C. New approach in vaginal prolapse repair: mini-invasive surgery associated with application of platelet-rich fibrin. Int Urogynecol J. 2012;23:715-22.
57. Runels C, Melnick H, Debourbon E, Roy L. A pilot study of the effect of localized injections of autologous platelet rich plasma (PRP) for the treatment of female sexual dysfunction. J Women's Health Care. 2014;3:169.
58. Amable PR, Carias RB, Teixeira MV, da Cruz Pacheco I, Correa do Amaral RJ, Granjeiro JM, et al. Platelet-rich plasma preparation for regenerative medicine: optimization and quantification of cytokines and growth factors. Stem Cell Res Ther. 2013;4:67.

14 CHAPTER

Managing Vaginismus with Botulinum Toxin: A Clinical Perspective

Bela Shah Jain, Naval Shah

INTRODUCTION

Vaginismus is a complex psychophysiological disorder characterized by involuntary contraction of the pelvic floor muscles, resulting in pain or difficulty during vaginal penetration. This can occur during sexual intercourse, gynecological examinations, or even the insertion of tampons. The condition is often associated with severe distress and can significantly impact a woman's sexual health, relationships, and overall quality of life. Though the exact prevalence is difficult to determine due to underreporting, it is estimated to affect between 1 and 7% of women globally.

Traditional treatments for vaginismus include psychosexual therapy, pelvic floor physical therapy, and vaginal dilator therapy. However, a subset of patients remains refractory to these interventions, continuing to experience significant discomfort and dysfunction. In recent years, botulinum toxin (BoNT) has emerged as a novel treatment option for such cases, offering a minimally invasive approach to relaxing the overactive pelvic floor muscles and restoring sexual function.[1,2] This chapter aims to provide a detailed clinical perspective on managing vaginismus with botulinum toxin, exploring its mechanism of action, procedural approach, efficacy, safety, and challenges.

PATHOPHYSIOLOGY OF VAGINISMUS

Vaginismus is typically classified into two types: *primary* and *secondary*. Primary vaginismus refers to cases where a woman has never been able to have penetrative intercourse due to pain or fear, often manifesting from a young age. Secondary vaginismus, on the other hand, develops later in life after a period of normal sexual function, potentially triggered by trauma, infections, surgeries, or psychological stressors.

The underlying pathophysiology involves both *psychological* and *physiological* factors. The psychological component often includes fear of pain (dyspareunia), sexual trauma, or anxiety disorders, while the physiological component centers on the *hypertonicity* or excessive tension of the pelvic floor muscles, specifically the levator ani, bulbospongiosus, and pubococcygeus muscles. These involuntary muscle contractions create a cycle of fear, pain, and avoidance, exacerbating the condition over time.

MECHANISM OF ACTION OF BOTULINUM TOXIN

Botulinum toxin, derived from the bacterium *Clostridium botulinum*, is a neurotoxin that blocks the release of acetylcholine at the neuromuscular junction.[3] By inhibiting acetylcholine, the toxin temporarily paralyzes muscle activity, leading to a reduction in spasm and hypertonicity.[4] In the context of vaginismus, BoNT specifically targets the overactive pelvic floor muscles, allowing them to relax and thereby facilitating pain-free vaginal penetration. The effects of the toxin typically last 3–6 months, during which time patients can undergo concurrent therapies, such as pelvic floor exercises and psychosexual counseling, to address the underlying causes of their condition.

This temporary muscle relaxation creates an ideal window for patients to retrain their pelvic muscles, gradually reducing the fear and pain associated with vaginal penetration. It is important to note, however, that while BoNT is highly effective in addressing the physiological component of vaginismus, it does not directly address the psychological factors, which often require concurrent cognitive-behavioral therapy (CBT) or sex therapy.

INDICATIONS FOR BOTULINUM TOXIN IN VAGINISMUS

Botulinum toxin is indicated in patients with *refractory vaginismus*, particularly those who have not responded to conventional treatments such as psychotherapy, pelvic floor physical therapy, or vaginal dilator use. It is especially beneficial in women whose vaginismus significantly impairs their quality of life, preventing them from engaging in sexual activity or even undergoing necessary gynecological examinations.[5]

In determining whether a patient is a suitable candidate for BoNT therapy, it is crucial to conduct a thorough assessment, including a detailed sexual history, psychological evaluation, and clinical examination to exclude other causes of dyspareunia, such as vulvodynia, endometriosis or pelvic inflammatory disease. Proper patient selection is key to achieving optimal outcomes with botulinum toxin.[6]

PROCEDURE

Administering botulinum toxin for the treatment of vaginismus is a relatively straightforward procedure, typically performed under conscious sedation, local anesthesia, or in some cases, general anesthesia if the patient experiences extreme anxiety or discomfort.

Patient Preparation

The patient is positioned in the lithotomy position. Conscious sedation or local anesthesia is administered to ensure comfort during the procedure.

For some women, the mere anticipation of the procedure may trigger muscle spasm, making the use of sedation a prudent choice. Deep sedation is to be avoided because some extent of muscle contraction is required to visualize the muscle for injecting the botulinum toxin.

Dosage

The dosage of BoNT-A can vary depending on the severity of the muscle hypertonicity. Most studies recommend starting with a dose of 100–200 units, divided across multiple injection sites within the pelvic floor.

Injection

About 100–200 units of botulinum toxin are diluted in 2 mL normal saline. Using a tuberculin syringe, it is injected submucosally in the bulbospongiosus muscle on the lateral sides sparing the anterior (suburethral) and posterior region to avoid the chances of urinary or anal incontinence respectively **(Fig. 1)**.

Postprocedure Care

After the injections, patients are typically observed for a short period to ensure there are no immediate adverse effects, and most are able to go home the same day. Vaginal dilator therapy is initiated immediately after the injection, helping to further retrain the muscles and prevent recurrence of the spasm **(Fig. 2)**.

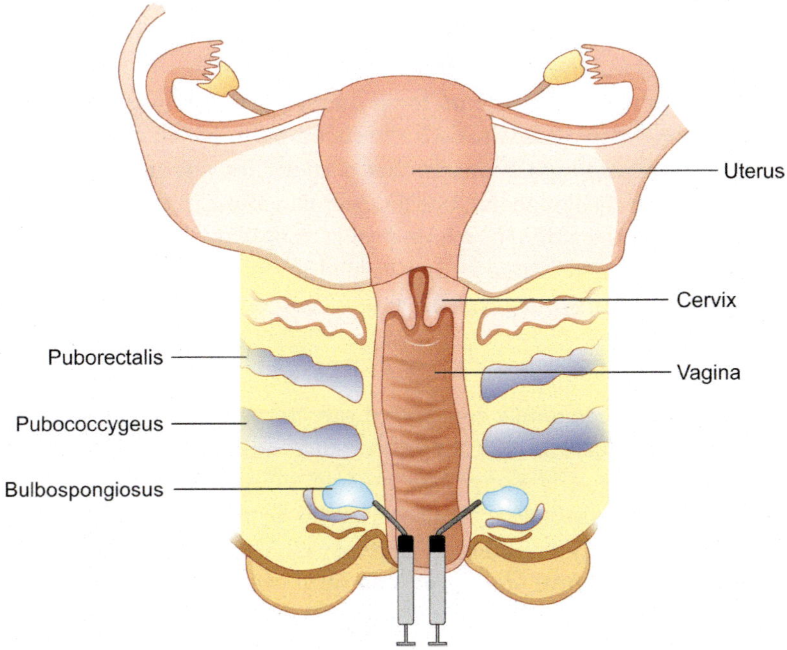

Fig. 1: Site of injection.

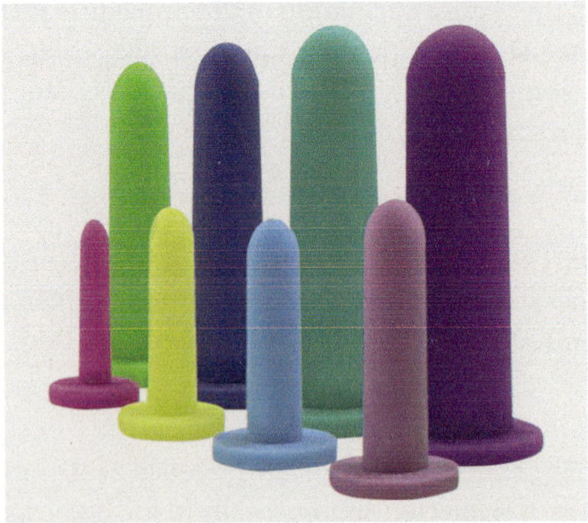

Fig. 2: Serial dilators used for vaginal dilator therapy.

EFFICACY AND CLINICAL OUTCOMES

Several studies in the last decade have demonstrated the efficacy of botulinum toxin in the treatment of vaginismus, with success rates ranging between 60 and 100%. In a 2020 randomized controlled trial by Pacik et al., 90% of patients reported significant improvement in their ability to achieve painless vaginal penetration following a single BoNT-A injection, combined with vaginal dilator therapy. Similar outcomes have been reported in other studies, with most patients experiencing a marked reduction in pain and improved sexual function within 2–4 weeks postinjection.

A key advantage of botulinum toxin therapy is that it allows patients to engage in penetrative activities with reduced pain, which can help break the cycle of fear and muscle spasm that perpetuates vaginismus. However, it is important to recognize that botulinum toxin alone may not be curative, particularly in cases where psychological factors play a dominant role. For this reason, multidisciplinary care, involving both physical therapy and psychotherapy, is recommended for optimal outcomes.

SAFETY PROFILE AND SIDE EFFECTS

Botulinum toxin is generally considered safe for use in the management of vaginismus. The most common side effects include local pain at the injection site, mild bruising, and temporary muscle weakness. In rare cases, the toxin may diffuse to adjacent muscles, potentially causing transient urinary incontinence or anal incontinence, but these effects are typically short-lived.

Compared to surgical options or long-term use of oral medications, botulinum toxin offers a minimally invasive option with a low risk of systemic side effects.

CHALLENGES AND CONSIDERATIONS

Despite its efficacy, several challenges and considerations must be addressed when using botulinum toxin for vaginismus management:[7]

Patient Selection

Successful outcomes with BoNT rely heavily on appropriate patient selection. Patients with primary vaginismus may require a more comprehensive and prolonged treatment plan compared to those with secondary vaginismus, where the condition developed after a period of normal sexual function.

Psychological Component

While botulinum toxin effectively relaxes the pelvic floor muscles, it does not address the underlying psychological factors associated with vaginismus. In many cases, the fear of pain or trauma persists even after muscle relaxation is achieved, necessitating ongoing psychosexual therapy.

CONCLUSION

Botulinum toxin is a promising treatment for women with refractory vaginismus, offering a minimally invasive option to relax hyperactive pelvic floor muscles and facilitate pain-free vaginal penetration. When combined with psychosexual therapy and pelvic floor rehabilitation, BoNT can significantly improve symptoms, enhance sexual function, and improve overall quality of life. However, success depends on proper patient selection and a multidisciplinary approach that addresses both the physical and psychological components of the condition.

REFERENCES

1. Pacik PT, Geletta S. Vaginismus treatment with Botox injections and progressive dilation under anesthesia: A 2-year follow-up study. J Sex Med. 2020;17(5):904-10.
2. Abdel-Hamid IA, Elrazek AE, Basha M, et al. Botulinum toxin-A for the treatment of refractory vaginismus: A prospective study. J Obstet Gynaecol Res. 2018;44(4):782-7.
3. Sobczak M, Kotarski J. Botulinum toxin type A in the treatment of vaginismus: A review of the current literature. Ginekol Pol. 2021;92(2):143-7.
4. Morin M, Khalifé S, Dubuc MJ, Bergeron S. Efficacy and safety of Botox injections for the treatment of provoked vestibulodynia: A randomized placebo-controlled trial. Am J Obstet Gynecol. 2017;216(1):41.e1-41.e9.
5. Thubert T, Faivre E, Naveau A, et al. Botulinum toxin A in the management of pelvic floor disorders. Int Urogynecol J. 2019;30(2):211-8.
6. Lee JS, Choi JB, Lee HS, et al. Long-term outcome of botulinum toxin type A injection for vaginismus. Obstet Gynecol Sci. 2022;65(3):268-74.
7. Shafik A, Shafik AA, El Sibai O, Shafik IA. Overactive pelvic floor syndrome: Role of botulinum toxin in its management. Clin Obstet Gynecol. 2016;59(3):539-45.

15

CHAPTER

Exosomes and Platelet-rich Plasma: Clinical Aspects in Cosmetic and Functional Gynecology

Rupinder Kaur Ruprai

INTRODUCTION

The field of cosmetic and functional gynecology is increasingly incorporating regenerative medicine to address a wide range of conditions. Exosomes and platelet-rich plasma (PRP) have emerged as powerful tools in this domain due to their ability to promote tissue regeneration, reduce inflammation, and enhance healing. These therapies have been used in vaginal rejuvenation, lichen sclerosus therapy, ovarian rejuvenation, and conditions affecting fertility, such as thin endometrium, endometriosis, and adenomyosis. Additionally, PRP and exosomes are increasingly combined with energy-based devices like fractional CO_2 lasers and radiofrequency to amplify their regenerative effects. This chapter explores the clinical aspects of exosomes and PRP in gynecology, focusing on vaginal rejuvenation, the O-Shot®, lichen sclerosus, ovarian rejuvenation, and improving infertility outcomes.

EXOSOMES IN FUNCTIONAL AND COSMETIC GYNECOLOGY

Mechanism of Action

Exosomes are small extracellular vesicles (30–150 nm) that mediate intercellular communication by transporting bioactive molecules such as proteins, lipids, and ribonucleic acid (RNA). Derived from mesenchymal stem cells (MSCs), exosomes possess potent regenerative properties, which include promoting angiogenesis, collagen synthesis, and modulating the immune response. Their ability to deliver these molecules to target cells without the risk of tumorigenesis makes them an attractive alternative to cell-based therapies like stem cells.[1]

Exosomes act by transferring their cargo of growth factors, cytokines, and microRNAs to damaged cells, thereby stimulating cellular repair and regeneration. This has important implications in gynecology, where tissue regeneration is crucial for conditions like vaginal atrophy, ovarian dysfunction, and endometrial abnormalities.

Clinical Applications

Vaginal Rejuvenation

Vaginal atrophy and dryness, particularly in postmenopausal women, lead to discomfort and sexual dysfunction. Exosomes have shown promise in rejuvenating vaginal tissues by promoting collagen production and improving tissue elasticity. A study by Zhuang et al. demonstrated that exosomes derived from MSCs significantly improved vaginal mucosa thickness, elasticity, and lubrication in a rat model of vaginal atrophy.[2] This suggests that exosomes could be an effective, noninvasive treatment for vaginal rejuvenation.

Ovarian Rejuvenation

Exosomes have also been explored for their potential in restoring ovarian function, particularly in women with diminished ovarian reserve (DOR) or premature ovarian failure (POF). Jiang et al. demonstrated that MSC-derived exosomes improved ovarian function by enhancing folliculogenesis and reducing local inflammation in an animal model. Their study showed that exosome therapy led to an increase in antral follicles and improved overall ovarian reserve.[3] These findings point to the possibility of exosome therapy being used for ovarian rejuvenation, which could benefit women with infertility due to poor ovarian reserve.

Endometriosis and Adenomyosis

Endometriosis and adenomyosis are chronic gynecological conditions characterized by abnormal growth of endometrial-like tissue outside the uterus (endometriosis) or within the uterine wall (adenomyosis). Both conditions are associated with chronic pain, heavy bleeding, and infertility. Exosomes derived from MSCs have shown anti-inflammatory and antifibrotic effects, making them a promising treatment for these disorders. Zhou et al. demonstrated that exosomes could reduce inflammation and fibrosis in animal models of endometriosis, potentially alleviating symptoms and reducing lesion size.[4] While human trials are needed, exosome therapy could offer a less invasive alternative to surgery for managing endometriosis and adenomyosis.

Poor Endometrium in Infertility

A thin endometrium is a significant cause of infertility, particularly in women undergoing assisted reproductive technologies (ARTs). Exosomes have shown promise in improving endometrial thickness and receptivity. Liang et al. found that MSC-derived exosomes promoted endometrial regeneration, increased vascularization, and improved pregnancy outcomes in a rat model with poor endometrium.[5] This suggests that exosomes could be used as an adjunct therapy to enhance endometrial quality and improve implantation rates in infertility treatments.

PLATELET-RICH PLASMA IN FUNCTIONAL AND COSMETIC GYNECOLOGY

Mechanism of Action

Platelet-rich plasma is an autologous concentrate of platelets, obtained by centrifuging the patient's blood. The concentrated platelets release growth factors such as platelet-derived growth factor (PDGF), vascular endothelial growth factor (VEGF), and transforming growth factor-beta (TGF-β), which are critical in tissue healing and regeneration.[6] PRP promotes angiogenesis, collagen production, and cellular proliferation, making it a powerful tool in treating gynecological conditions.

Clinical Applications

Vaginal Rejuvenation

Platelet-rich plasma has been successfully used in vaginal rejuvenation to improve tissue elasticity, lubrication, and overall sexual satisfaction. A study by Kamolpornwijit et al. demonstrated that PRP injections led to significant improvements in vaginal lubrication, elasticity, and sexual health in postmenopausal women experiencing vaginal atrophy.[7] PRP's ability to enhance collagen synthesis and improve tissue hydration makes it an effective treatment for restoring vaginal function in women with menopausal symptoms.

O-Shot® for Sexual Function

The O-Shot® is a PRP-based treatment designed to improve female sexual function and treat conditions like stress urinary incontinence (SUI). PRP is injected into the vaginal and clitoral regions to enhance tissue sensitivity, increase blood flow, and promote collagen production. Runels et al. showed that women who received the O-Shot® reported enhanced sexual satisfaction, improved orgasmic function, and increased vaginal lubrication.[8] The O-Shot® is gaining popularity as a nonsurgical option for women seeking to improve their sexual health and treat SUI.

Lichen Sclerosus

Lichen sclerosus is a chronic inflammatory condition that affects the vulva, causing thinning of the skin, itching, and pain. PRP has shown potential in treating lichen sclerosus by reducing inflammation and promoting tissue repair. Taverna et al. conducted a study in which patients with lichen sclerosus received PRP injections. The results showed a significant reduction in symptoms, improvement in skin texture, and better overall quality of life.[9] PRP offers a noninvasive treatment option for this debilitating condition, with minimal side effects and long-lasting results.

COMBINED USE OF PRP AND EXOSOMES WITH ENERGY-BASED DEVICES

Mechanism of Action

Energy-based devices such as fractional CO_2 lasers and radiofrequency are widely used in gynecology to promote tissue remodeling and improve vaginal elasticity. These devices work by creating controlled microthermal damage, which triggers the body's natural healing processes, including collagen production and tissue repair. When PRP or exosome therapy is combined with energy-based devices, the regenerative effects are significantly enhanced, leading to faster and more comprehensive tissue healing.[10]

Clinical Applications

Vaginal Rejuvenation

The combination of PRP or exosomes with fractional CO_2 lasers or radiofrequency devices has been shown to produce superior results in vaginal rejuvenation. Salvatore et al. demonstrated that women who received fractional CO_2 laser therapy combined with PRP injections reported greater improvements in vaginal elasticity, lubrication, and overall satisfaction compared to those who underwent laser therapy alone.[11] The synergistic effect of these therapies enhances collagen production and accelerates tissue regeneration, offering long-lasting improvements in vaginal health.

Lichen Sclerosus

Lichen sclerosus can also benefit from the combined use of energy-based devices with PRP or exosome therapy. Fractional CO_2 lasers and radiofrequency treatments stimulate collagen remodeling and tissue regeneration, while PRP or exosomes enhance healing by providing growth factors and promoting cellular repair. Clinical studies have shown that this combination leads to more significant symptom relief and better long-term outcomes in patients with lichen sclerosus.[12]

Ovarian Rejuvenation

Ovarian rejuvenation using PRP or exosomes is an emerging area of interest, particularly for women with diminished ovarian reserve (DOR) or premature ovarian failure (POF). PRP injections into the ovarian cortex aim to stimulate folliculogenesis, restore ovarian function, and improve fertility outcomes.

In a study by Sfakianoudis et al., PRP injections were used in women with DOR, resulting in restored ovarian function and spontaneous pregnancies in some cases.[13] Similarly, exosomes derived from MSCs have shown the ability to improve ovarian function by modulating the ovarian microenvironment, reducing inflammation, and promoting follicular growth.[3] These therapies offer a promising alternative to traditional fertility treatments for women with reduced ovarian function.

Endometriosis and Adenomyosis

PRP and exosomes have shown promise in managing endometriosis and adenomyosis, both of which are characterized by chronic inflammation and fibrosis. The growth factors in PRP and the anti-inflammatory properties of exosomes can reduce fibrosis and promote tissue regeneration in affected areas. Zhou et al. demonstrated that MSC-derived exosomes reduced inflammation and fibrosis in animal models of endometriosis, suggesting that exosomes could be a viable therapeutic option for this condition.[4] PRP has also been explored for its potential to promote healing and reduce pain in women with endometriosis and adenomyosis.

Poor Endometrium in Infertility

A thin endometrium is a major cause of infertility and implantation failure in women undergoing ART. Both PRP and exosomes have been investigated for their ability to improve endometrial thickness and receptivity. PRP injections into the endometrium have been shown to increase endometrial thickness, improve blood flow, and enhance implantation rates in women with refractory thin endometrium. Zadehmodarres et al. found that intrauterine PRP injections significantly improved endometrial thickness and pregnancy outcomes in women undergoing ART.[14] Similarly, exosomes have shown promise in promoting endometrial regeneration and improving fertility outcomes in animal models.[5]

CONCLUSION

Exosomes and PRP are emerging as powerful tools in cosmetic and functional gynecology, offering innovative solutions for conditions such as vaginal atrophy, lichen sclerosus, ovarian dysfunction, and infertility related to thin endometrium. These therapies promote tissue regeneration, reduce inflammation, and enhance overall healing, making them valuable in both therapeutic and cosmetic applications. Additionally, combining exosomes or PRP with energy-based devices has shown enhanced clinical outcomes, particularly in vaginal rejuvenation and lichen sclerosus therapy. As research continues to evolve, exosomes and PRP are expected to play an increasingly important role in gynecological care, providing noninvasive options for women seeking improved reproductive health and quality of life.

REFERENCES

1. Kalluri R, LeBleu VS. The biology, function, and biomedical applications of exosomes. Science. 2020;367(6478):eaau6977.
2. Zhuang M, Chen X, Duan X, et al. Mesenchymal stem cell-derived exosomes promote the regeneration of atrophic vaginal mucosa in a rat menopause model. Stem Cell Res Ther. 2020;11(1):234.
3. Jiang Z, Hu X, Yu H, et al. MSC-derived exosomes improve ovarian function and increase follicle reserves in a premature ovarian failure mouse model. Stem Cell Res Ther. 2021;12(1):128.
4. Zhou Q, Wang T, Zha S, et al. Role of exosomes in the pathogenesis of endometriosis. Fertil Steril. 2020;113(6):1215-21.
5. Liang Y, Duan L, Xiong J, Zhu W. Exosomes derived from mesenchymal stem cells repair injured endometrium and improve fertility in a rat model. Stem Cell Res Ther. 2019;10(1):106.
6. Marx RE. Platelet-rich plasma (PRP): What is PRP and what is not PRP? Implant Dent. 2001;10(4):225-8.
7. Kamolpornwijit W, Manchana T, Thanapprapasr D, et al. Efficacy of autologous platelet-rich plasma injections in the treatment of vaginal atrophy: A prospective pilot study. J Obstet Gynaecol Res. 2020;46(8):1302-8.
8. Runels C, Benson J, Castellano K. The use of platelet-rich plasma in aesthetic facial rejuvenation and sexual enhancement: A review. Aesthet Surg J. 2020;40(1).
9. Taverna G, Di Meo S, Giusti G, et al. Autologous platelet-rich plasma for the treatment of vulvar lichen sclerosus. Med Hypotheses. 2018;121:107-9.
10. Gambacciani M, Palacios S. Laser therapy for the restoration of vaginal function. Maturitas. 2017;99:10-5.
11. Salvatore S, Nappi RE, Zerbinati N, Calligaro A, Ferrero S, Origoni M, et al. A 12-week treatment with fractional CO_2 laser for vulvovaginal atrophy: A pilot study. Climacteric. 2014;17(4):363-9.
12. Vicari M, Di Martino M, Nardelli GB, et al. Use of autologous platelet-rich plasma in the treatment of stress urinary incontinence. Urologia. 2021;88(1):13-8.
13. Sfakianoudis K, Simopoulou M, Nitsos N, et al. Autologous platelet-rich plasma treatment enables pregnancy for a woman in premature menopause. J Clin Med. 2018;7(10):188.
14. Zadehmodarres S, Heidar Z, Ebrahimi M. Intrauterine infusion of autologous platelet-rich plasma in women undergoing assisted reproduction: A pilot study. J Reprod Infertil. 2017;18(4):388-92.

16 CHAPTER

Stem Cells and Gynecology

Poonam Mishra

INTRODUCTION

Stem cells have emerged as a promising therapeutic tool in various medical fields, including gynecology. Their ability to differentiate into multiple cell types and self-renew makes them invaluable in both regenerative medicine and disease treatment.[1]

TYPES OF STEM CELLS

Stem cells can be broadly categorized into two main types: embryonic stem cells (ESCs) and adult stem cells.

Embryonic Stem Cells

Source: Derived from the inner cell mass of blastocysts, which are early-stage embryos.

Potency: Pluripotent, meaning they can differentiate into any cell type in the body.

Usage in gynecology: ESCs hold potential in treating infertility by generating viable eggs or supporting uterine regeneration. However, their use is limited due to ethical concerns.

Adult Stem Cells

Unlike ESCs, adult stem cells are found in various tissues and organs throughout life and have more restricted differentiation potential. They are typically multipotent, meaning they can differentiate into several but not all cell types.[2]

Source: Found in tissues such as bone marrow, adipose tissue, and reproductive organs.

Potency: Multipotent, limited to producing cell types from a specific tissue or organ.

Subtypes of Adult Stem Cells

- *Hematopoietic stem cells (HSCs):* Found in the bone marrow and responsible for generating blood cells.
- *Mesenchymal stem cells (MSCs):* Found in various tissues, including bone marrow, adipose tissue, and the placenta. They can differentiate into bone, cartilage, muscle, and fat cells.
- *Endometrial stem cells:* Found in the lining of the uterus, capable of regenerating the endometrial tissue, and play a crucial role in endometrial repair during each menstrual cycle.
- *Ovarian stem cells:* Present in the ovaries, potentially involved in follicular development and fertility preservation.[3]

APPLICATIONS OF STEM CELLS IN GYNECOLOGY

Stem cells have shown promising potential in various aspects of gynecology, primarily focusing on regenerative medicine and infertility treatments. Below are some key applications:

- *Treatment of endometriosis:* Endometrial stem cells can potentially be used to restore normal tissue function in women with endometriosis.
- *Regeneration of uterine lining:* Endometrial stem cells may help regenerate damaged or thin uterine linings in cases of Asherman's syndrome or infertility due to thin endometrium.[4]
- *Ovarian regeneration:* Ovarian stem cells hold promise in treating premature ovarian failure or age-related infertility by promoting ovarian function.[5]
- *Treatment of pelvic organ prolapse:* Mesenchymal stem cells (MSCs) have been explored for their ability to strengthen pelvic tissues and support the repair of damaged pelvic structures.
- *Fertility preservation:* Stem cell-based therapies might help women undergoing cancer treatment preserve their fertility by regenerating ovarian tissue.[6]
- *Menstrual disorders:* By harnessing the regenerative potential of endometrial stem cells, researchers are investigating new treatments for disorders such as menorrhagia and amenorrhea.[7]

CONCLUSION

Stem cells offer a wide array of potential applications in gynecology, from treating infertility to regenerating reproductive tissues. While embryonic stem cells are powerful, their use is limited due to ethical issues. Adult stem cells, particularly mesenchymal and endometrial stem cells, present significant potential for therapeutic applications in women's health. Further research is needed to fully realize the clinical potential of stem cell therapy in gynecology.

REFERENCES

1. Abbot JD, Liang Q. Stem cells in reproductive biology and medicine. Nat Rev Mol Cell Biol. 2016;17(5):324-36.
2. Gargett CE, Masuda H. Adult stem cells in the endometrium. Mol Hum Reprod. 2010;16(11):818-34.
3. Mansouri N, Saleki A. Ovarian stem cells and their role in fertility preservation: A systematic review. J Assist Reprod Genet. 2018;35(6):915-26.
4. Mardia AR, Deane JA. Mesenchymal stem cells in gynecological regenerative medicine: Current status and future directions. Hum Reprod Update. 2020;26(1):44-64.
5. Niknejad H, Yazdanpanah G, Zare-Shahneh A. Stem cells in female reproductive biology and regenerative medicine. Stem Cells Dev. 2013;22(18):2415-24.
6. Donnez J, Dolmans MM. Fertility preservation in women. N Engl J Med. 2017;377(17):1657-65.
7. Zhang D, Lu Y. Endometrial stem cells: Role in uterine biology and disease. Front Endocrinol. 2019;10(123):1-10.

17

CHAPTER

Neovagina: Techniques, Innovations, and Future Directions

Manjula Anagani, Sindura Gadde

INTRODUCTION

Neovaginoplasty, or the creation of a neovagina, is primarily indicated for patients with congenital vaginal agenesis, such as Mayer-Rokitansky-Küster-Hauser (MRKH) syndrome, a condition characterized by the absence of the uterus and upper vaginal canal. This condition occurs in 1 in 5,000 to 1 in 10,000 female births. It significantly affects both reproductive function and psychological well-being, necessitating an approach that addresses physical, aesthetic, and functional outcomes. Recent developments in surgical materials, techniques, and technologies aim to offer improved results with fewer complications **(Figs. 1A and B)**.

INDICATIONS FOR NEOVAGINA CONSTRUCTION

- Congenital anomalies, such as MRKH syndrome, where the vagina and uterus are underdeveloped.
- Gender-affirming surgery for transgender women.
- Postsurgical or traumatic loss, such as after pelvic exenteration.

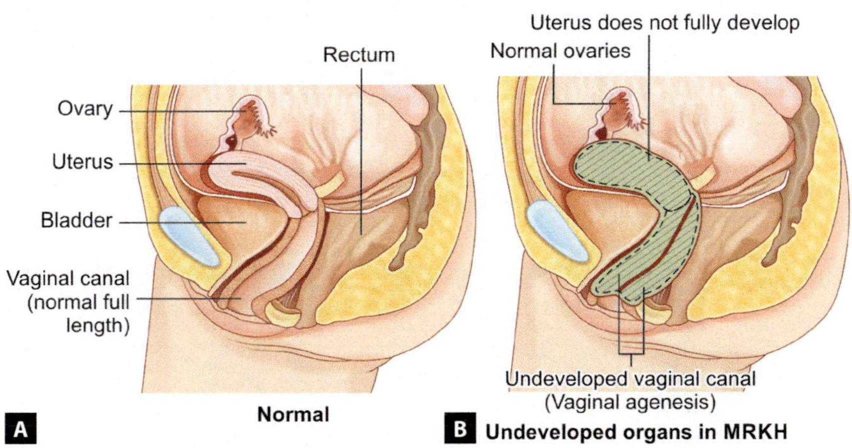

Figs. 1A and B: Normal, undeveloped organs in Mayer-Rokitansky-Küster-Hauser (MRKH).

TECHNIQUES OF NEOVAGINOPLASTY

Nonsurgical Techniques

- Pressure dilatation methods:
  - Frank technique—intermittent pressure technique
  - Ingrams—modification of intermittent pressure technique

Techniques such as the Frank and Ingram methods use vaginal dilators to gradually expand a shallow vaginal dimple. This approach requires patient motivation and consistent effort, often for months, to achieve a functional vaginal canal. It remains a first-line, noninvasive treatment recommended before considering surgery.

Success rates and limitations: Though effective in some cases, pressure dilation can be time-consuming and may not produce satisfactory results in patients with more severe vaginal agenesis **(Figs. 2A and B)**.

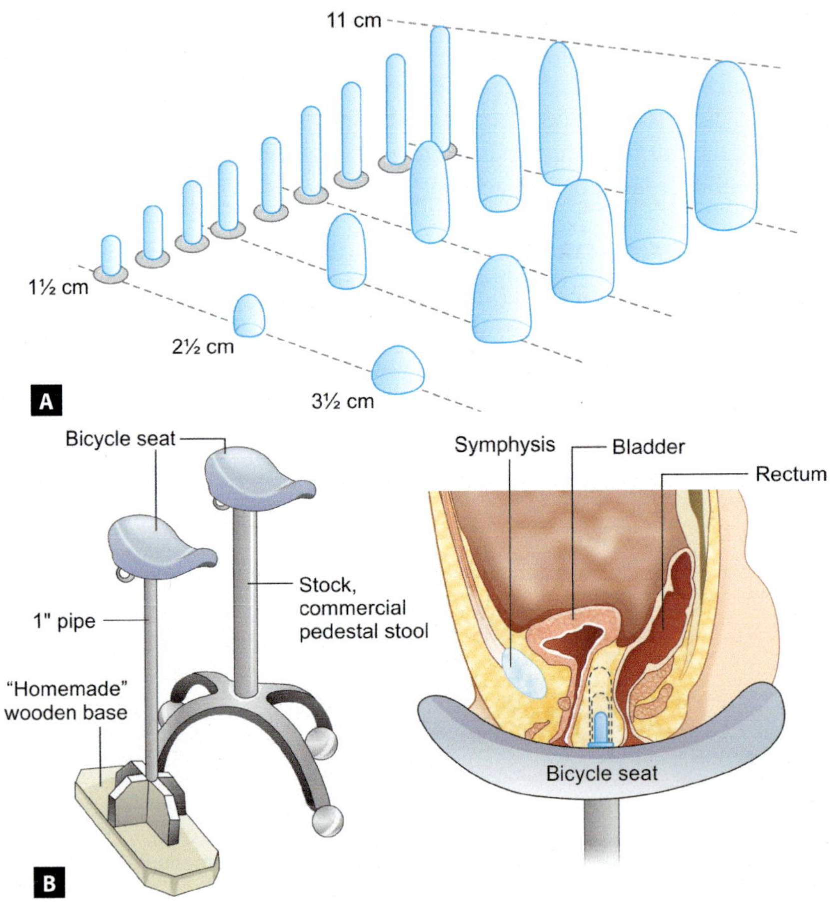

Figs. 2A and B: Clear, lucite, graduated dilators used in Frank and Ingram methods.

Surgical Techniques

- Timing of these procedures—when the patient attains full growth, is psychologically prepared, and is socially and/or sexually mature
  - Higher estrogen levels are present—preventing stenosis
  - Patient can perform dilatation herself
  - Ideal time—after 18 years of age.
- *McIndoe technique:* Involves creating a vaginal canal and lining it with a split-thickness skin graft. While effective, this approach poses risks such as donor site morbidity and graft contraction. Additionally, the need for multiple procedures may affect patient quality of life **(Fig. 3)**.
- *Modifications of McIndoe technique:* Using various adhesion barriers like peritoneum, skin flaps, amnion, buccal mucosa and bowel (colon)
- *Vecchietti procedure:* A minimally invasive laparoscopic method that involves the gradual traction of a device through the abdomen to create a neovagina. It requires hospitalization and has shown good long-term anatomical and functional results. However, it can cause discomfort due to the traction device and requires patient compliance **(Figs. 4 and 5)**.
- *Davydov procedure:* Uses peritoneal tissue to create a neovagina, typically performed laparoscopically. It has become popular due to its minimal donor site morbidity and the potential for spontaneous lubrication of the neovagina **(Figs. 6A to N)**.
- *A Novel Anagani approach in neovaginoplasty:* Using intercede. The use of Interceed (oxidized regenerated cellulose) as a barrier material in neovaginoplasty has gained popularity due to its unique properties:

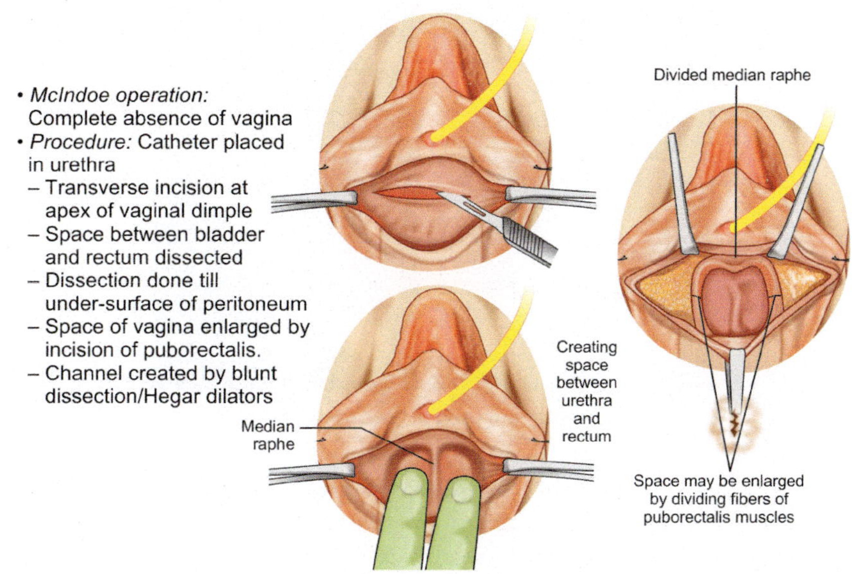

Fig. 3: McIndoe technique

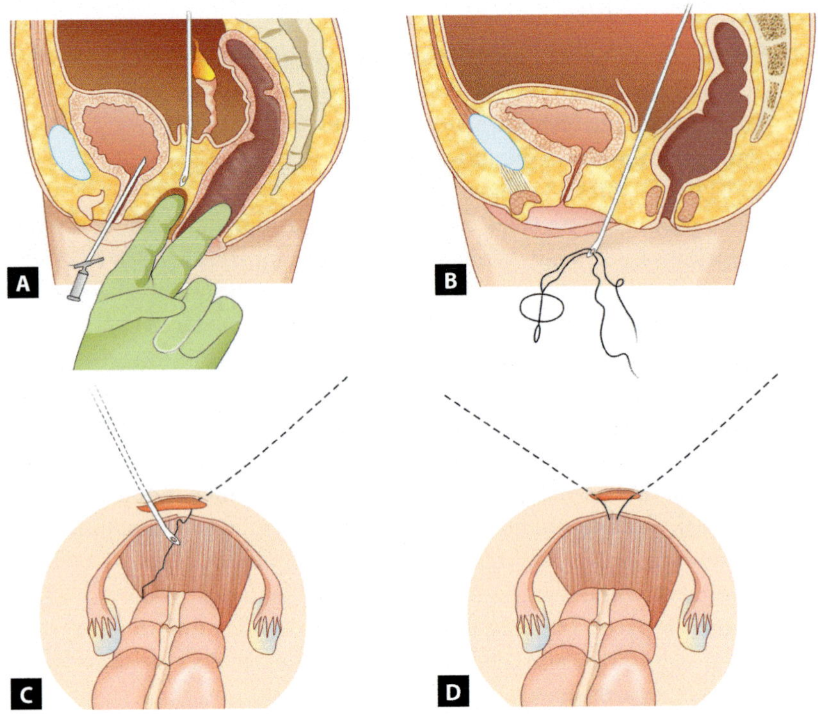

Figs. 4A to D: Vecchietti procedure.

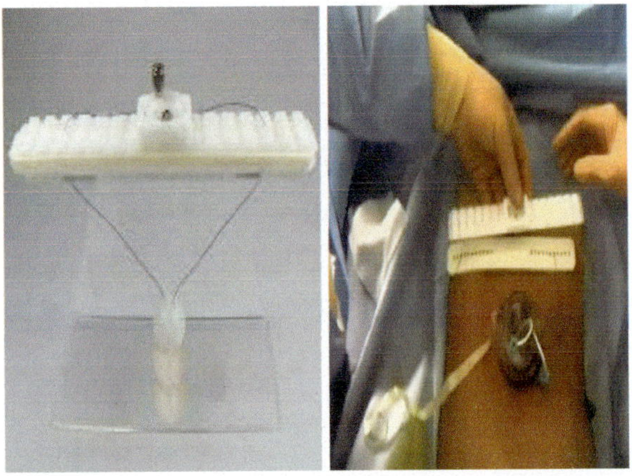

Fig. 5: Instrument used in Vecchietti procedure.

- *Mechanism:* Interceed, an oxidized regenerated cellulose, acts as an absorbable adhesion barrier, forms a gelatinous mass which acts as a protective coating on raw surfaces, allowing re-epithelialization to occur under it with no risk of infectious transmission.

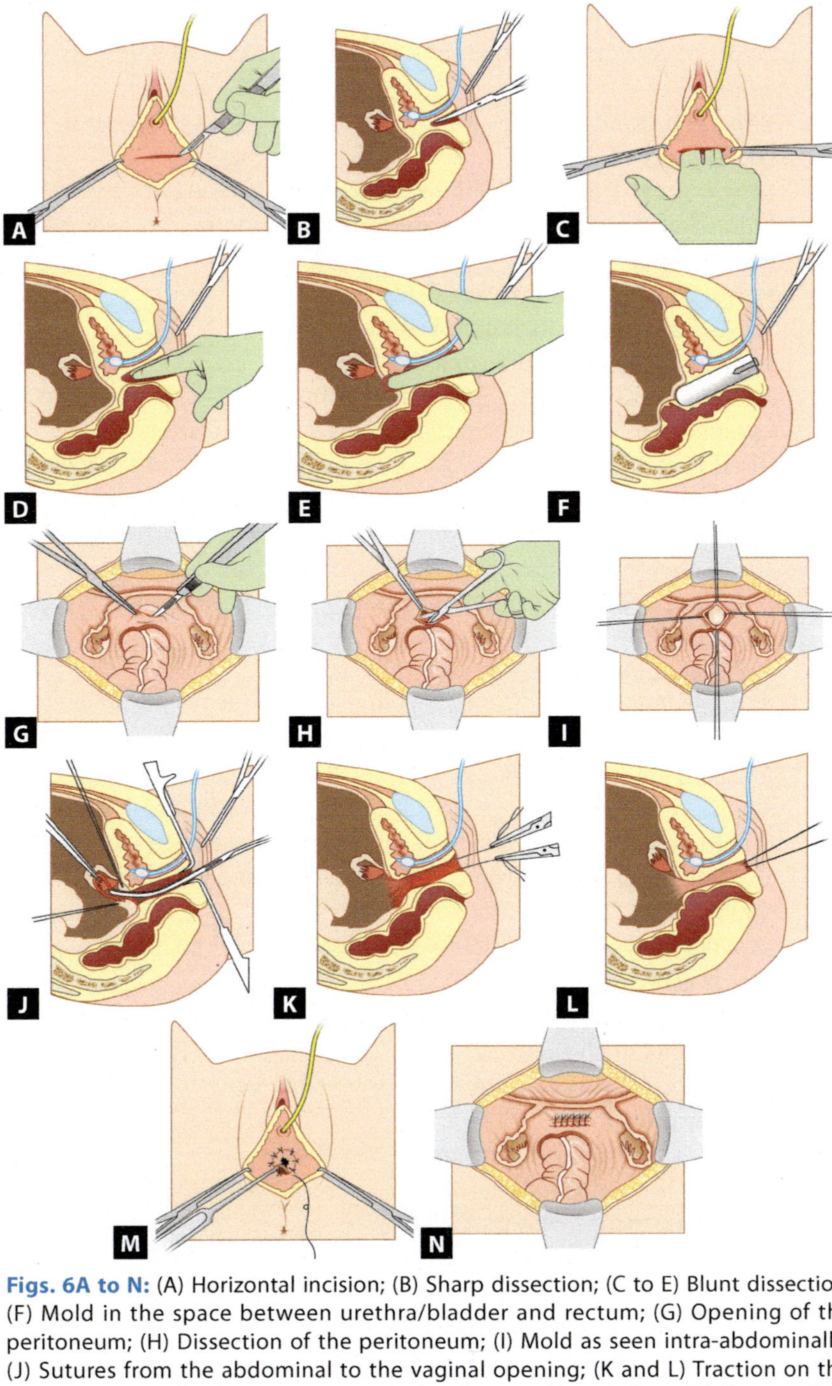

Figs. 6A to N: (A) Horizontal incision; (B) Sharp dissection; (C to E) Blunt dissection; (F) Mold in the space between urethra/bladder and rectum; (G) Opening of the peritoneum; (H) Dissection of the peritoneum; (I) Mold as seen intra-abdominally; (J) Sutures from the abdominal to the vaginal opening; (K and L) Traction on the peritoneum; (M) The peritoneum is sutured to the vaginal epithelium; (N) Closure of the abdominal peritoneum.

This prevents adhesion between the vaginal mold and surrounding tissues, allowing for complete squamous epithelialization of the neovagina.

- *Advantages:*
  - The technique reduces operative time (typically around 15–20 minutes)
  - Lowers the risk of complications such as graft-related infections
  - Eliminates the need for donor site surgery or another procedure like laparoscopy
    - No need for another? Plastic surgeon
    - No permanent scar at donor site/operative site
    - Technically less challenging

Studies show a neovaginal length of approximately 8.5–9 cm at 6 months, with a high rate of patient satisfaction regarding sexual function.

- *Challenges:* Although promising, complications such as stenosis or occasional granulation tissue formation may still occur, requiring additional interventions. Moreover, the technique's success heavily relies on postoperative care, including the use of vaginal molds and dilators.
- *Procedure:* Under GA, in a lithotomy position (with buttocks over hanging over the table), prophylactic antibiotic to be given.
  - *On local examination:* Vaginal dimple noticed
  - The space between the bladder and urethra in front and rectum behind was dissected up to the pelvic peritoneum
  - 9–10 cm length and 4–5 cm width of space created using modified shears technique after 25 cc of diluted vasopressin is instilled. (Dilution—20 units in 200 mL of NS). Hemostasis is secured.
  - Vaginal edges are in turned and sutured at 4 angles using 3-0 rapid Vicryl
  - Mold is created using middle or thumb finger of no. 8/8.5 surgical gloves and Vaseline gauze
  - Interceed is placed on the whole of mold and the mold with Interceed is inserted into the neovagina.
  - Labia minora was sutured with 3 interrupted sutures using silk 2-0 keeping mold in situ.
  - Total OR time is approximately 15–20 minutes
- *Postprocedure course:*
  - Catheterized for 7 days post surgery.
  - Complete bed rest and liquid diet for 4 days followed by soft diet for 3 days.
  - Regular betadine dressing to be done.
  - Mobilized on day 4.
  - Mold is removed on day 7 and thorough irrigation of vagina done with normal saline.

- Neovagina formed is healthy with good epithelialization.
- Taught to use dilators with estrogen gel, three times a day for 10 minutes each time, for good epithelialization.
- Discharged on day 8 in stable condition
- Postoperative checks are advised at 4 weeks, 6 weeks, 2 months, quarterly and then half yearly.
- Every visit—vaginal depth, degree of epithelialization are to be examined

- *Laparoscopic and combined approaches:* Laparoscopic techniques have transformed neovaginoplasty by providing minimally invasive access to pelvic structures. Procedures like the laparoscopic Vecchietti or Davydov methods utilize small abdominal incisions to create a neovagina, resulting in quicker recovery, less pain, and improved cosmetic outcomes. Combining laparoscopic techniques with biomaterials like Interceed or SIS grafts enhances the surgical process by reducing complications associated with open surgeries.

Emerging Alternatives

- *3D-printed vaginal molds:* Personalized 3D-printed molds made from biocompatible materials are being explored to customize the shape and size of the neovagina based on individual anatomy. This approach may further enhance patient outcomes by providing better-fitting molds and reducing the need for subsequent interventions.
- *Synthetic scaffolds:* Innovations in tissue engineering include the use of synthetic or biodegradable scaffolds seeded with autologous cells, promoting tissue regeneration and integration. While still experimental, these methods show promise for future neovaginoplasty applications.

ADDRESSING LONG-TERM OUTCOMES

Long-term follow-up is essential to evaluate the durability of neovaginoplasty results.

Factors such as sexual function, neovaginal maintenance, and psychological well-being need to be monitored. The success rate is often gauged using the Female Sexual Function Index (FSFI), with recent studies reporting improved scores in lubrication, orgasm, and overall satisfaction postneovaginoplasty.

COMPLICATIONS AND MANAGEMENT

Common complications after neovaginoplasty include:

- *Stenosis:* Often managed with periodic dilations.
- *Granulation tissue formation:* May require chemical cautery or surgical excision.

- *Fistula formation:* Rare but can occur, especially in complex cases with underlying conditions like MRKH syndrome.
- *Postoperative pain:* Typically managed with analgesics and gradual return to normal activities

PSYCHOLOGICAL SUPPORT AND MULTIDISCIPLINARY CARE

Patients undergoing neovaginoplasty often face psychological challenges related to body image and sexual identity. A multidisciplinary approach involving gynecologists, psychologists, and physical therapists ensures comprehensive care. Postsurgical counseling and support groups can help address concerns and promote positive outcomes.

FUTURE DIRECTIONS AND INNOVATIONS

Emerging techniques include tissue engineering and stem cell therapy for neovagina creation. These methods hold promise for improving the quality and functionality of neovaginas with fewer complications.

CONCLUSION

Vaginal agenesis involves issues of physical abnormality, body image, sexual identity and sexual/reproductive functioning. Requires long-term medical and psychological management.

Neovaginoplasty has advanced significantly, moving toward less invasive and more patient-centered approaches. Techniques using Interceed and other novel biomaterials have shown to be effective and safe, offering an alternative to traditional methods:

- The use of Interceed in surgical vaginoplasty is shown to give encouraging results
- *Interceed* rapidly forms a gelatinous mass—acts as protective coating on raw surfaces—allowing re-epithelialization to occur under it
- Interceed—relatively inexpensive, readily available and biodegradable
- Interceed requires no preparation and no risk of infectious transmission
- Safe and effective minimally invasive procedure which does not require any separate surgery
- OR times are considerably decreased
- Least morbidity and comparable outcomes

While emerging technologies such as 3D-printed molds and synthetic scaffolds hold promise for further improvements, careful patient selection and individualized treatment planning remain crucial for optimal results.

As research continues, the goal will be to refine these techniques to provide better quality of life for individuals with vaginal agenesis.

SUGGESTED READING

1. ACOG Committee Opinion No. 728. Surgical Options for Vaginal Agenesis. Obstet Gynecol. 2017;129(5):e177-e182.
2. Bouman MB, et al. Intestinal vaginoplasty: a feasible and safe technique in gender-affirming surgery. J Sex Med. 2016;13(5):999-1005.
3. Buncamper ME, et al. Surgical techniques for vaginoplasty in male-to-female transsexuals. BJU International. 2017;119(3):330-8.
4. Callens N, De Cuypere G, De Sutter P, Monstrey S, Weyers S, Piet Hoebeke, et al. An update on surgical and non-surgical treatments for vaginal hypoplasia. Hum Reprod Update. 2014;20(5):775-801.
5. Creatsas G, Deligeoroglou E, Makrakis E, Kontoravdis A, Papadimitriou L. Creation of a neovagina following Williams vaginoplasty and the Creatsas modification in 111 patients with Mayer-Rokitansky-Küster-Hauser syndrome. Fertil Steril; 2001;76(5):1036-40.
6. Davydov SN, Zhvitiashvili OD. Formation of the vagina by intestinal transplantation. Soviet Surg. 1974;10:23-7.
7. Deffieux X, et al. Surgical complications of neovagina construction in patients with Mayer-Rokitansky-Küster-Hauser syndrome. J Minim Invasive Gynecol. 2011;18(4):483-90.
8. Ethicon, Inc. Premarket approval. [online] Available at:www.accessdata.fda.gov/scripts/cdrh/cfdocs/cfpma/pma.cfm?id=P880047....
9. Gupta S, Hurwitz DJ. Surgical approaches for vaginal reconstruction. Plast Reconstr Surg. 2007;120(7):1570-81.
10. Hensle TW, Reiley EA. Surgical options for vaginoplasty. Curr Urol Rep. 1998;1(2):157-64.
11. HS Moon, et al. Simple neovaginoplasty using spontaneous regeneration ability of labial and vestibular flap in patients with Müllerian agenesis. Gynecol Minim Invasive Ther; 2017.
12. Jackson ND, Rosenblatt PL. Use of Interceed absorbable adhesion barrier for vaginoplasty. Obstet Gynecol. 1994;84(6):1048-50.
13. JM. Ingram the bicycle seat stool in the treatment of vaginal agenesis and stenosis: a preliminary report. Am J Obstet Gynecol. 1981;140(8):867-73.
14. Laufer MR, et al. "Vaginal reconstruction: a review of surgical techniques and complications. J Pediatr Adolesc Gynecol. 2002;15(1):29-35.
15. McIndoe A. The treatment of congenital absence and obliterative conditions of the vagina. Br J Plast Surg. 1950;2(4):254-67.
16. Morcel K, Camborieux L, Guerrier D. Mayer-Rokitansky-Küster-Hauser (MRKH) syndrome. Orphanet J Rare Dis. 2007;2:13.
17. Motoyama S, Laoag-Fernandez JB, Mochizuki S, Yamabe S, Maruo T. Vaginoplasty with Interceed absorbable adhesion barrier for complete squamous epithelialization in vaginal agenesis. Am J Obstet Gynecol; 2003.
18. Raya-Rivera AM, Esquiliano D, Fierro-Pastrana R, López-Bayghen E, Valencia P, Ordorica-Flore R, et al. Tissue-engineered autologous vaginal organs in patients: A pilot cohort study. Lancet. 2014;384(9940):329-36.
19. RT, Frank. The formation of an artificial vagina without operation. Am J Obstet Gynecol; 1938.

20. Schneider M, et al. Regenerative medicine and neovagina construction: a comprehensive review. J Gynecol Surg. 2020;36(2):68-75.
21. Spert H. Historical development of the concept of vaginal reconstruction. Am J Obstet Gynecol. 1950;60(5):1135-41.
22. Söhn C, et al. Long-term results of neovaginal reconstruction: an analysis of surgical and psychosocial outcomes. J Plast Reconstr Aesthet Surg. 2015; 68(3):398-405.
23. Vatsa R, Bharti J, Roy KK, Kumar S, Sharma JB, Singh N, et al. Evaluation of amnion in creation of neovagina in women with Mayer-Rokitansky-Kuster-Hauser syndrome. Fertil Steril. 2017;108(2):341-5.

18

CHAPTER

Vulval Skin Lightening and Brightening

Savana Chongtham

INTRODUCTION

Vulval skin lightening and brightening is a growing trend within the field of cosmetic gynecology and intimate aesthetics. These procedures are aimed at addressing hyperpigmentation and uneven skin tone in the vulval region, which can result from several factors such as hormonal changes, aging, friction, and inflammation. The rising interest in vulval aesthetics parallels the demand for other cosmetic procedures aimed at enhancing the appearance of intimate areas, reflecting broader social and cultural factors that emphasize body image and self-confidence.

CAUSES OF VULVAL HYPERPIGMENTATION

- *Hormonal changes:* Hormonal fluctuations during puberty, pregnancy, or menopause can lead to increased melanin production. Estrogen and progesterone increase the sensitivity of melanocytes, which leads to darkening of the skin in sensitive areas like the vulva.[1]
- *Friction:* Repeated friction caused by tight clothing, shaving, or prolonged sitting can contribute to irritation and postinflammatory hyperpigmentation (PIH).
- *Inflammation:* Conditions such as lichen sclerosus, eczema, and recurrent infections can trigger an inflammatory response, which often leads to skin darkening as part of the healing process.
- *Aging:* Over time, skin loses elasticity, and melanin production becomes less regulated, contributing to a darker appearance.
- *Ethnicity and genetics:* Individuals with darker skin tones (Fitzpatrick skin types IV-VI) are naturally more prone to hyperpigmentation due to a higher baseline melanin content.[2]

COMMON APPROACHES TO VULVAL SKIN LIGHTENING

Vulval skin lightening and brightening can be achieved through a variety of techniques, ranging from topical agents to advanced laser therapies.

Each approach targets melanin production and distribution within the skin, although the mechanisms and safety profiles differ.

Topical Agents

Hydroquinone: Hydroquinone is a well-established depigmenting agent used for the treatment of hyperpigmentation. It works by inhibiting tyrosinase, the enzyme responsible for melanin production. However, its use in sensitive areas such as the vulva is controversial due to the risk of irritation and ochronosis, a condition where the skin darkens paradoxically.[3]

Azelaic acid: Azelaic acid is a naturally occurring dicarboxylic acid with anti-inflammatory and depigmenting properties. It is considered a safer alternative to hydroquinone, especially for sensitive skin areas like the vulva. Its mode of action includes the inhibition of DNA synthesis in hyperactive melanocytes.[4]

Kojic acid: Derived from fungi, kojic acid has been employed as a skin-lightening agent. It works by inhibiting tyrosinase, though its effectiveness is generally considered milder compared to hydroquinone. Kojic acid is often included in combination therapies to enhance its efficacy while minimizing side effects.[5]

Niacinamide: This form of vitamin B_3 reduces melanin transfer from melanocytes to keratinocytes, which helps to lighten skin. Its anti-inflammatory properties also make it suitable for managing postinflammatory hyperpigmentation in delicate regions.[6]

Chemical Peels

Chemical peels involve the application of exfoliating agents to remove the superficial layers of the skin, promoting cell turnover and reducing pigmentation. Mild peels such as *glycolic acid* and *lactic acid* are commonly used in intimate areas for their gentle yet effective exfoliating properties. They help in brightening the skin by enhancing the penetration of lightening agents and promoting regeneration of new skin cells. However, care must be taken to avoid burns or irritation due to the sensitivity of the vulval region.

Laser and Energy-based Treatments

Laser treatments have become popular for intimate skin lightening due to their precision and effectiveness. The following are commonly used technologies:

Fractional CO_2 lasers: These lasers work by creating microinjuries in the skin, which stimulates collagen production and accelerates skin renewal. They are particularly useful for lightening hyperpigmented areas, though multiple sessions are required for optimal results.[7]

Q-switched Nd

Lasers: Nd lasers target melanin with high-intensity pulses of light, breaking down pigment clusters in the skin. This method is considered safe for use on darker skin tones, where other treatments may be less effective or increase the risk of hypopigmentation.[8]

Intense pulsed light (IPL): IPL is a nonlaser light therapy that can treat pigmentation by delivering broad-spectrum light to the affected area. While it is less aggressive than laser therapy, it can still lead to noticeable improvement in skin tone after several sessions.

SAFETY AND EFFICACY CONCERNS

While the demand for vulval skin lightening continues to grow, there are concerns about the safety and long-term efficacy of these treatments. The vulval skin is particularly sensitive, and interventions in this area carry a higher risk of complications such as burns, irritation, allergic reactions, and scarring.

- *Overuse of topical agents:* Prolonged or inappropriate use of topical depigmenting agents such as hydroquinone can lead to adverse effects like ochronosis, paradoxical hyperpigmentation, or skin thinning. Hence, the use of these agents should be closely monitored by a healthcare provider.
- *Postlaser complications:* Laser treatments, if performed incorrectly, can result in burns, scarring, or changes in texture. Patients with darker skin tones are particularly at risk for postinflammatory hypopigmentation or hyperpigmentation following laser therapy, making it crucial to select the appropriate laser type and settings.

ETHICAL CONSIDERATIONS

The rise in demand for vulval skin lightening raises important ethical questions. The normalization of such procedures may reinforce unrealistic beauty standards and contribute to body image dissatisfaction. Some critics argue that these procedures are unnecessary and potentially harmful, as they often stem from societal pressures rather than medical necessity.

Furthermore, the promotion of vulval lightening treatments may disproportionately affect women of color, who are more likely to experience hyperpigmentation due to their skin type.

PATIENT EDUCATION AND COUNSELING

Given the sensitive nature of vulval lightening procedures, patient education and counseling are crucial. Patients should be informed about the realistic outcomes of treatment, the potential risks, and the need for maintenance therapy. It is also important to manage expectations, as complete depigmentation is often unrealistic, especially in individuals with darker skin tones.

CONCLUSION

Vulval skin lightening and brightening represent a growing sector in cosmetic gynecology. While there are a variety of treatment options available, ranging from topical agents to laser therapies, each method carries its own risks and benefits. Healthcare providers must prioritize patient safety, ensure ethical practice, and engage in thorough patient counseling to ensure that individuals are making informed decisions based on personal preferences rather than societal pressures.

REFERENCES

1. Palumbo A, d'Ischia M, Misuraca G, Prota G. Mechanism of inhibition of melanogenesis by hydroquinone. Biochim Biophys Acta. 1991;1073(1):85-90.
2. Taylor SC, Cook-Bolden F, Rahman Z, Sills MR. Defining skin of color. J Am Acad Dermatol. 2006;54(5 Suppl 2).
3. Vashi NA, de Castro Maymone MB, Kundu RV. Aging differences in ethnic skin. J Clin Aesthet Dermatol. 2016;9(1):31-8.
4. Del Rosso JQ, Levin J. The clinical relevance of maintaining the integrity of the stratum corneum in acne vulgaris. J Clin Aesthet Dermatol. 2011;4(9):22-42.
5. Lim JT. Treatment of melasma using kojic acid in a gel containing hydroquinone and glycolic acid. Dermatol Surg. 1999;25(4):282-4.
6. Hakozaki T, Minwalla L, Zhuang J, Chhoa M, Matsubara A, Miyamoto K, et al. The effect of niacinamide on reducing cutaneous pigmentation and suppression of melanosome transfer. Br J Dermatol. 2002;147(1):20-31.
7. Alster TS, Tanzi EL. Improvement of facial and neck skin texture and laxity with a nonablative fractional resurfacing device. Dermatol Surg. 2004;30(4 Pt 1):508-12.
8. Wanner M, Tanzi E. Fractional photothermolysis for photoaging of the hands. Dermatol Surg. 2007;33(5):539-42.

19 CHAPTER

Ovarian Rejuvenation

Preeti Jindal, Neharika Malhotra, Sumitu Sahdev, Muskan Mittal

BACKGROUND

Longevity of life has increased. With it the desire of woman to postpone her childbearing has also increased. Simultaneously, the time a woman spends in peri- and postmenopausal phase is more than 30 years. This has led to search for new methods to retain ovarian function, postpone menopause and regenerate the aging oocytes. Let's read in this chapter what all advances have taken place in this direction.

INTRODUCTION

It was believed that women are born with a fixed reserve of eggs, which starts getting depleted from the time they are born. At birth a female has close to 1–2 million eggs and by the time she achieves puberty they are left with only 25–30% of her original reserve that is around 300,000–400,000. This pool slowly gets depleted until the time she achieves menopause by the age of 45–50 years. It is also important to appreciate that thousands of senescent eggs still persist even at the inception of perimenopause. These eggs may have a potential to be activated and hence may result in follicular growth, fertilization, pregnancy, and live birth.

Aging of the female reproductive system is directly associated with disruption of ovarian function and jeopardizes fertility potential, ultimately leading to menopause—a stage identified hitherto as irreversible.[1-3] The ovary in a female's body, has very important reproductive and endocrine roles.[4] In today's era, females planning a pregnancy in their 30s and 40s has increased exponentially, the problem of diminished ovarian reserve (DOR) is rampant and bringing into light various strategies which can help these females produce their own genetic offspring.

There are currently few therapy options available to help women with their ovarian reserve and oocyte quality like coenzyme Q10, dehydroepiandrosterone, vitamins including vitamins C and D, or dietary or supplement isoflavones. No study has categorically validated the routine administration of these bioactive substances. Normally most of the females with low ovarian reserve will need artificial reproductive techniques such as intrauterine insemination (IUI), in vitro fertilization (IVF), oocyte donation program, surrogacy, and also adoption in some cases.

Ovarian platelet-rich plasma (PRP) is a newly developing technique that uses PRP to stimulate the ovaries and improve female fertility. Platelet-rich plasma is produced by centrifugation and separation of its various components from patient's own blood, which contains plasma (55%), red blood cells (41%), platelets, and white blood cells (4%). Red blood cells are removed during the centrifugation and separation process, and plasma is created with a 5–10 times higher concentration of growth factors.[5,6] Alpha granules, which are found in platelets in PRP, produce a variety of substances that promote angiogenesis, cell proliferation, and growth.[7] Specific growth factors and cytokines include transforming growth factor-beta, fibroblast growth factor, insulin-like growth factors 1 and 2, vascular endothelial growth factor, and epidermal growth factor are released[8] **(Fig. 1)**.

When injected into the ovaries, PRP releases these growth factors, which can stimulate cellular rejuvenation, improve ovarian blood flow, and promote the recruitment and maturation of healthy eggs, thereby naturally and effectively enhancing the fertility.[9] Studies have shown PRP has a positive effect on survival and growth of follicles.[10] A case series has also shown biochemical pregnancy following autologous PRP intraovarian infusion.[11] Also, there have been reports of livebirths in poor responder patients following autologous PRP intraovarian infusion.[12] To ascertain whether autologous intraovarian PRP injection is advantageous in female reproduction, particularly for women with poor ovarian response (POR), primary ovarian insufficiency (POI), and early menopause, it needs to be researched on a larger scale in a clinical trial setting with standardized preparation, injection, and follow-up techniques.

Ovarian rejuvenation using PRP is not a cure for infertility, but it can be a helpful option for women who are struggling to conceive due to very low

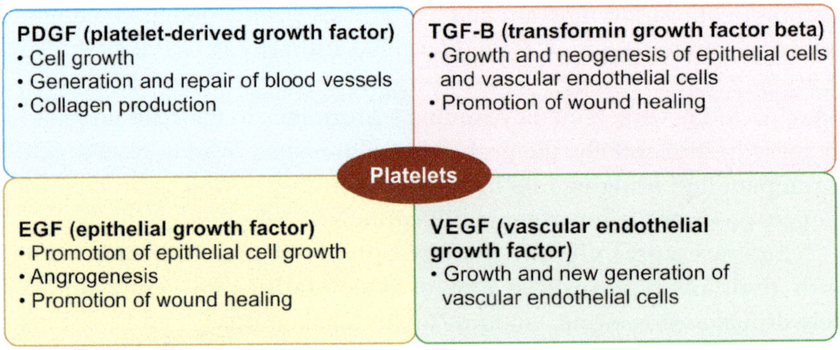

Fig. 1: Growth factors released by platelets.
Source: Annals of Burns and Fire disasters, Vol. XXV-n. 4-December 2012.

anti-Müllerian hormone (AMH) and poor ovarian reserve. It is a safe and desirable option for many couples as there is no need to go for donor eggs. The procedure is generally safe and well-tolerated, and it can be performed on an outpatient basis.

INDICATIONS FOR OVARIAN PLATELET-RICH PLASMA

- Menopausal or perimenopausal women on 50 years
- Infertile women >35 years having low egg reserve and low AMH levels
- Women with premature ovarian failure
- Primary ovarian insufficiency
- Loss of ovarian function due to chemotherapy
- Ovarian dysfunction

CONTRAINDICATIONS FOR OVARIAN PLATELET-RICH PLASMA

- Acute infectious or systemic diseases
- Viral hepatitis B and C
- Allergic reactions to anticoagulants
- Immunosuppressive conditions
- Blood clotting disorders
- Pregnancy and lactation
- Mental disorders
- History of oncology
- Age under 18 years **(Fig. 2)**

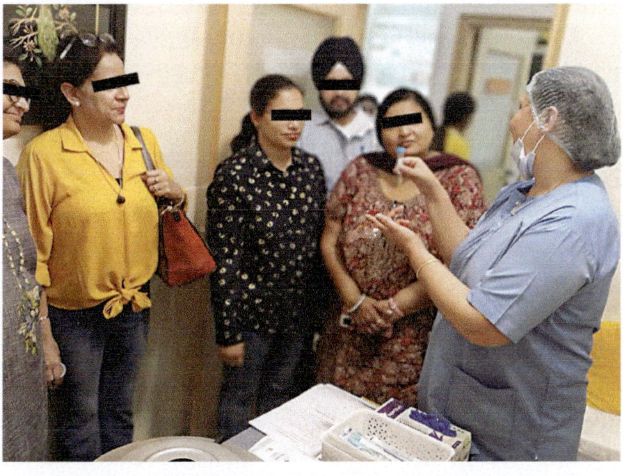

Fig. 2: Platelet-rich plasma (PRP) preparation procedure being demonstrated to the candidates for cosmetic gyne course.

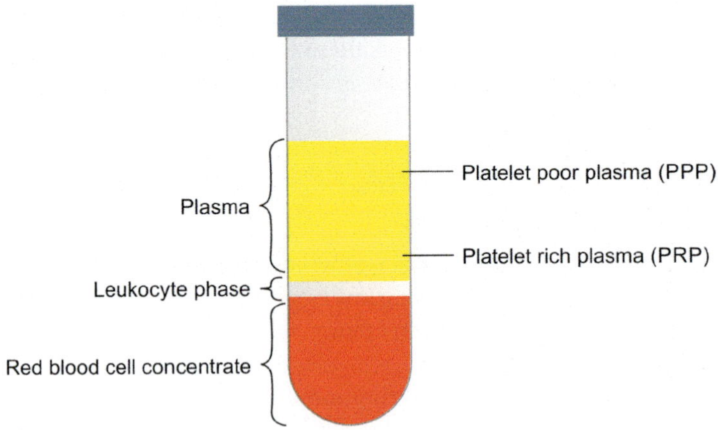

Fig. 3: Different fractions obtained after centrifugation of anticogulated blood.

PLATELET-RICH PLASMA PREPARATION PROCEDURE

Platelet-rich plasma is prepared by differential centrifugation process. About 10–15 mL of venous blood is obtained by venipuncture in ACDA (acid citrate dextrose solution A) prefilled syringe. The blood is not chilled at any time before or during platelet separation. The ideal temperature during centrifugation is 21–24°C. Centrifuge the blood using a "soft spin" at 1,200 rpm for 12 minutes. Three layers are formed because of its density. The bottom layer consisting of red blood cells (RBCs), the middle layer having platelets and white blood cells (WBCs) and the top platelet poor plasma layer. The top and middle layer are transferred to an empty sterile tube and centrifuged at a higher speed of 3,300 rpm for 7 minutes (a hard spin) to obtain platelet concentrate. The lower one-third is PRP and upper two-thirds is platelet poor plasma (PPP). PPP is discarded and PRP is now ready for injection[11,12] **(Fig. 3)**.

PLATELET-RICH PLASMA INSTILLATION PROCEDURE

For ovarian rejuvenation, we require 4 mL (2–2 mL, each ovary) so dilution of the pellet is done accordingly. Patient is subjected to day-care total intravenous anesthesia. Once the PRP is prepared and activated, it is filled in the egg retrieval needle, so as to remove any air which is present in the channel of the needle. A 17-gauge single lumen needle is usually employed, moving across from the peripheral to central part of the ovary and forth, carefully covering the distance from one side to the other. Activated PRP is then introduced via a syringe attached to the transvaginal probe transducer. Once the channel is filled with PRP and all the air is removed, transvaginal ultrasonography (TVUS) probe is inserted in the vagina, the ovary is visualized

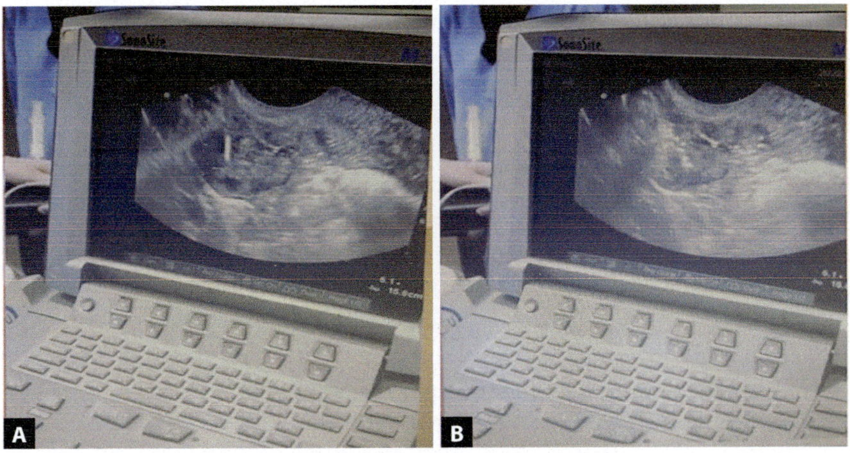

Figs. 4A and B: Ovarian platelet-rich plasma (PRP) instillation procedure being performed at The Touch Clinic, Mohali.

and the needle is inserted through the biopsy guide needle attached to the TVUS probe and then into the ovary under ultrasonography guidance. Extreme caution is exercised so as to avoid penetrating the outer wall of the ovary into the peritoneal cavity. 2 mL PRP is injected into each ovary at two or three sites. The duration of the intraovarian injection procedure is in the range of approximately 4–7 minutes.

For patients, whose ovaries are too small and felt inaccessible by the TVUS, a laparoscopic instillation of PRP is done into both the ovaries. For these patients the blood is taken on admission to the hospital, after which, they are prepared for and subjected to a therapeutic hysterolaparoscopy wherein the visualization of the small ovaries becomes much easier and the instillation of PRP was done by the egg retrieval needle inserted through the ancillary 5 mm trocar where it can be injected at the hilum of the ovaries. The laparoscopic approach was chosen in order to get a better judgment about the instillation, it gives precise location and opportunity to check whether it is leaking. While performing sonography the leakage cannot be checked, and there is a difficulty in making out the hilum of ovaries. Moreover, when done laparoscopically, identifying other factors like any deformity in the uterus or endometriosis can be checked easily **(Figs. 4A and B)**.

Postprocedure care: After the PRP injections, the patient is monitored for a short period to ensure that there are no immediate complications or adverse reactions.

Follow-up: Follow-up appointments help to monitor response to the treatment, assess changes in ovarian response and evaluate the need for additional cycles of ovarian rejuvenation.

The number of sessions needed for ovarian rejuvenation therapy with PRP can vary from patient to patient. The major factors to be considered for deciding the number of sessions often depend on the patient's age, current ovarian reserve, response to treatment. Since PRP therapy for ovarian rejuvenation is still an evolving technique, there is no standardized protocol regarding the number of sessions.

The time taken for ovarian rejuvenation therapy with PRP to start acting can vary from patient to patient and the exact timeline is still being studied. In general, it may take several weeks for the effects of ovarian rejuvenation with PRP to become apparent. This is because the PRP is intended to stimulate and regenerate ovarian tissue and ovarian germ cells, which may require time for cellular changes and tissue repair to occur.

The two tests done commonly to assess ovarian reserve are AMH and transvaginal sonography for antral follicle count (AFC). After 4–6 weeks, if ovarian rejuvenation has been effective, there will be an increase in AFC and AMH values indicating an improvement in the ovarian reserve.

RISKS AND SIDE EFFECTS

Ovarian PRP is a safe and minimally invasive procedure. The primary risks or side effects are minor discomfort, bruising, or spotting after the procedure. The complications, such as postprocedural pain, bleeding, hematoma formation, are negligible. Allergies, hypersensitivity reactions, or anesthesia-related complications are rarely observed. It has been hypothesized that PRP promotes the development of isolated human primordial and primary follicles to the preantral stage.[13] Studies have revealed that autologous intraovarian infusion of PRP with considerable amount of growth factors and cytokines has shown to enhance ovarian regeneration as well as reactivation of folliculogenesis[14] and has led to new horizons of hope in the field of reproductive gynecology.

ADVANTAGES OF PLATELET-RICH PLASMA THERAPY FOR OVARIAN REJUVENATION

- *Higher antral follicles:* Chances of retrieving more number of mature oocytes after ovarian stimulation during an IVF cycle.
- *Higher AMH values:* Chances of improving AMH values, indicative of improved ovarian reserve.
- *Spontaneous resumption of menstrual cycles* in women with premature menopause.
- *Improvement in ICSI/IVF cycle outcome:* In poor responders with increased number and quality of oocytes leading to better embryos.
- *Higher number of retrieved oocytes in IVF cycle* resulting in higher and better quality of embryos in IVF cycle.

OTHER BENEFITS OF PLATELET-RICH PLASMA

The benefits of PRP will continue to be seen as they are used in more areas in the medicine for regenerative procedures.[15] PRP is a safe and effective alternative treatment modality in patients with stress urinary incontinence.[16,17]

Regarding the timing between ovarian rejuvenation and ovarian stimulation for IVF, there is no standard consensus or established guideline. However, at least 6 weeks gap should be given between ovarian PRP injection and ovarian stimulation for IVF. Patients should take multivitamins and antioxidants during this period.

CONCLUSION

Ovarian rejuvenation by autologous intraovarian infusion of PRP can be one of the newer potential treatments to restore the reproductive and endocrine functions of the ovary, which can help a female conceive and reproduce her own genetic offspring and avert the possibility of using a donor program for the same. Though, this procedure has given us good results but multiple studies with different geographic populations and more robust data would be required to stamp an affirmative and build an overall positive consensus for this procedure. Stem cell therapies are under research and have also been used for ovarian rejuvenation, however, data are not yet available to show its enhanced therapeutic effects. Further studies are required to evaluate its efficacy.

REFERENCES

1. Leidal AM, Levine B, Debnath J. Autophagy and the cell biology of age-related disease. Nature Cell Biology. 2018;20:1338-48.
2. Hamet P, Tremblay J. Genes of aging. Metabolism. 2003;52:5-9.
3. Finch CE. The menopause and aging, a comparative perspective. J Steroid Biochem Mol Biol. 2014;142:132-41. Fufa D, Shealy B, Jacobson M, et al. Activation of platelet-rich plasma
4. Faddy MJ. Follicle dynamics during ovarian ageing. Mol Cell Endocrinol. 2000;163:43-8.
5. Sills ES, Wood SH. Autologous activated platelet-rich plasma injection into adult human ovary tissue: molecular mechanism, analysis, and discussion of reproductive response. Bioscience Reports. 2019;39(6):BSR20190805.
6. Dhurat R, Sukesh MS. Principles and methods of preparation of platelet-rich plasma: a review and author's perspective. J Cutan Aesthet Surg. 2014;7:189-97.
7. Pavlovic V, Ciric M, Jovanovic V, Stojanovic P. Platelet-rich plasma: A short overview of certain bioactive components. Open Med (Wars). 2016;11(1):242-7.
8. Marx RE. Platelet-rich plasma (PRP): what is PRP and what is not PRP? Implant Dent. 2001;10(4):225-8.
9. Seckin S, Ramadan H, Mouanness M, Kohansieh M, Merhi Z. Ovarian response to intraovarian platelet-rich plasma (PRP) administration: hypotheses and potential mechanisms of action. J Assist Reprod Genet. 2022;39(1):37-61.

10. Sills ES, Rickers NS, Li X, Palermo GD. First data on in vitro fertilization and blastocyst formation after intraovarian injection of calcium gluconate-activated autologous platelet rich plasma. Gynecol Endocrinol. 2018;34(9):756-60.
11. Everts PA, Mahoney CB, Hoffmann JJ, Schönberger JPAM, Box HAM, van Zundertet A, et al. Platelet-rich plasma preparation using three devices: implications for platelet activation and platelet growth factor release. Growth Factors. 2006;24(3):165-71.
12. Sfakianoudis K, Simopoulou M, Nitsos N, Rapani A, Pantou A, Vaxevanoglou T, et al. A case series on platelet-rich plasma revolutionary management of poor responder patients. Gynecol Obstet Invest. 2019;84(1):99-106.
13. Hosseini L, Shirazi A, Naderi MM, Shams-Esfandabadi N, Boroujeni SB, Sarvari A, et al. Platelet-rich plasma promotes the development of isolated human primordial and primary follicles to the preantral stage. Reprod Bio Med Online. 2017;35(4):343-50.
14. Anitua E, Andia I, Ardanza B, Nurden P, Nurden AT. Autologous platelets as a source of proteins for healing and tissue regeneration. Thromb Haemost. 2004;91(01):4-15.
15. Jindal P. Aesthetic and Regenerative Gynaecology by Springer; 2022. [online] Available from https://doi.org/10.1007/978-981-16-1743-0 [Last accessed December, 2024].
16. Jindal P, Sahdev S, Gulati R, Kundal I. Nonsurgical management of stress urinary incontinence (SUI). Acta Sci Women's Health. 2020;2(11):51-4.
17. Jindal P. Aesthetic, Regenerative and Cosmetic Gynecology by Jaypee Brothers; 2025. [online] Available from https://jaypeebrothers.com/products/9781787791848 [Last accessed December, 2024]

20 CHAPTER

Regenerative Therapies for Thin Endometrium: PRP, Stem Cells, Exosomes, and Other Approaches

Jaideep Malhotra, Narendra Malhotra, Keshav Malhotra, Neharika Malhotra

INTRODUCTION

Thin endometrium is a significant challenge in reproductive medicine, often associated with poor reproductive outcomes, such as implantation failure, recurrent miscarriage, and decreased success rates in assisted reproductive technology (ART). Conventional therapies, including hormonal treatments and endometrial scratching, often have limited efficacy. Recently, regenerative therapies like platelet-rich plasma (PRP) antioxidants, no-donors (Larginene), aspirin, heparin, sildenafil, stem cells, exosomes, and other novel approaches have emerged as promising alternatives. These therapies aim to enhance endometrial thickness, improve vascularization, and create a more receptive endometrial environment.[1]

PLATELET-RICH PLASMA

Platelet-rich Plasma for Endometrial Regeneration

- *Treatment of thin endometrium:* PRP has been used to treat thin endometrium, which is a common cause of implantation failure in IVF. PRP injections into the uterine cavity can improve endometrial thickness, enhance blood flow, and increase the expression of implantation-related markers, leading to better reproductive outcomes.
- *Asherman's syndrome:* PRP has shown promise in treating Asherman's syndrome, characterized by intrauterine adhesions. PRP promotes the regeneration of endometrial tissue, reduces fibrosis, and restores a receptive endometrium.[2]

Ovarian Rejuvenation and Infertility

- *Premature ovarian insufficiency (POI):* PRP is being explored as a treatment to rejuvenate ovarian function in women with POI. PRP injections into the ovarian cortex can stimulate follicular development, improve hormonal levels, and enhance fertility potential.

- *Age-related ovarian decline:* PRP therapy is considered a potential option to enhance ovarian reserve in older women, improving the quantity and quality of oocytes and potentially delaying the onset of menopause.

  PRP is derived from autologous blood and contains a high concentration of platelets and growth factors. These components promote tissue regeneration, angiogenesis, and anti-inflammatory effects, making PRP a valuable treatment option for thin endometrium.
- *Mechanism of action:* PRP releases growth factors such as platelet-derived growth factor (PDGF), transforming growth factor-beta (TGF-β), and vascular endothelial growth factor (VEGF). These factors enhance cell proliferation, differentiation, and angiogenesis, improving endometrial thickness and receptivity.
- *Clinical evidence:* Studies have demonstrated that intrauterine infusion of PRP can significantly increase endometrial thickness and improve pregnancy outcomes in patients with thin endometrium. A recent meta-analysis reported that PRP treatment increased endometrial thickness by an average of 1.5 mm and improved clinical pregnancy rates by 30–50% in ART cycles.
- *Protocol and administration:* PRP is typically prepared by centrifugation of the patient's blood and then infused into the uterine cavity, usually on days 10–12 of the menstrual cycle. Repeat administrations may be required, depending on individual responses. Newer approach of hysteroscopic subendometrial injection is showing better results.

STEM CELL THERAPY

Stem cells are undifferentiated cells with the unique ability to self-renew and differentiate into various specialized cell types. The most commonly used stem cells in clinical practice include:

- *Mesenchymal stem cells (MSCs):* Derived from bone marrow, adipose tissue, umbilical cord, and other sources, MSCs have shown great promise in gynecological regenerative medicine due to their ability to modulate inflammation, promote tissue repair, and enhance angiogenesis.
- *Embryonic stem cells (ESCs):* Derived from the inner cell mass of blastocysts, ESCs can differentiate into any cell type but are limited by ethical concerns and risks of tumorigenicity.
- *Induced pluripotent stem cells (iPSCs):* These are adult cells reprogrammed to an embryonic-like state, offering the potential to create patient-specific cells without the ethical issues associated with ESCs.
- *Endometrial stem cells (EnSCs):* Stem cells derived from the endometrial lining show potential in regenerative gynecology due to their high proliferation rate and ease of accessibility.

Endometrial Regeneration and Infertility Treatments

- *Thin endometrium:* MSCs have been used to treat thin endometrium, a condition that leads to infertility due to poor endometrial receptivity. Stem cell therapy can enhance endometrial thickness, improve blood flow, and promote a more favorable environment for embryo implantation.
- *Asherman's syndrome:* Characterized by intrauterine adhesions, Asherman's syndrome can cause severe infertility. MSCs and EnSCs have shown promise in breaking down adhesions and regenerating normal endometrial tissue, significantly improving reproductive outcomes.

Ovarian Regeneration and Reproductive Aging

- *Premature ovarian insufficiency (POI):* Stem cell therapies are being explored to rejuvenate ovarian function in women with POI. MSCs can promote follicular development, improve hormonal balance, and restore fertility potential in affected individuals.
- *Age-related ovarian decline:* Stem cell interventions aim to delay ovarian aging and enhance ovarian reserve, offering potential treatments for women seeking fertility preservation later in life.

Stem cells offer a unique regenerative potential due to their ability to differentiate into various cell types and secrete bioactive factors that aid tissue repair.

- *Types of stem cells used:*
  - *Bone marrow-derived stem cells (BMDSCs):* Known for their regenerative properties, BMDSCs can differentiate into endometrial cells and promote tissue remodeling.
  - *Menstrual blood-derived stem cells (MenSCs):* MenSCs are easily accessible and exhibit high proliferative capacity. They have shown promising results in regenerating damaged endometrium and improving its thickness.
  - *Adipose-derived stem cells (ADSCs):* ADSCs are rich in mesenchymal stem cells (MSCs) and are known to enhance angiogenesis and cell proliferation in the endometrial lining.
- *Clinical evidence:* Recent trials indicate that stem cell therapy can lead to increased endometrial thickness and improved live birth rates. A study by Zhao et al. (2022) demonstrated that autologous MenSCs increased endometrial thickness by 2.0–3.0 mm in women with Asherman's syndrome and chronic endometritis, significantly enhancing fertility outcomes.
- *Administration protocols:* Stem cells are typically injected into the uterine cavity under ultrasound guidance. The number of injections may vary depending on the severity of the thin endometrium. The newer approach of subendometrial, hysteroscopic-guided injection is showing better results.

EXOSOMES

Therapeutic applications: Exosomes are emerging as a novel therapeutic approach due to their ability to deliver molecular cargo directly to target cells, offering potential treatments for conditions where conventional therapies are limited.[3]

- *Regenerative medicine:* Exosomes derived from mesenchymal stem cells (MSCs) have demonstrated regenerative properties in treating endometrial thinning, Asherman's syndrome, and pelvic floor disorders. They promote angiogenesis, reduce fibrosis, and enhance tissue repair.
    - *Endometrial regeneration:* MSC-derived exosomes have been shown to enhance endometrial cell proliferation, reduce fibrosis, and improve implantation rates in cases of thin endometrium, offering a potential therapy for patients with recurrent implantation failure.
    - *Pelvic floor disorders:* Exosome therapy is being explored to repair pelvic floor tissues, providing a nonsurgical approach to managing conditions such as urinary incontinence and pelvic organ prolapse.

Exosomes are small extracellular vesicles released by cells that play a critical role in cell-to-cell communication, transferring proteins, lipids, and RNA molecules that can influence cellular behavior.

- *Mechanism of action:* Exosomes derived from MSCs or other regenerative cells contain bioactive molecules that modulate inflammation, promote angiogenesis, and enhance tissue regeneration. Their ability to deliver therapeutic cargo to target cells makes them an innovative treatment for thin endometrium.
- *Clinical evidence:* Preclinical studies have shown that exosomes can improve endometrial regeneration in animal models of thin endometrium by enhancing angiogenesis and reducing fibrosis. Emerging clinical data suggest potential benefits in human subjects, but large-scale trials are still needed.
- *Administration:* Exosomes can be delivered intrauterine through infusions. Further research is ongoing to optimize their delivery and dosing strategies. Subendometrial hysteroscopic-guided injection is also under trial. Exosomes are commercially available and have to be reconstituted before injection.

OTHER REGENERATIVE THERAPIES

- *Growth factor therapy:* Direct administration of growth factors like VEGF and granulocyte-colony stimulating factor (G-CSF) has shown some promise in improving endometrial thickness, though results are inconsistent and depend on individual patient profiles.
- *Hyaluronic acid:* Used as a scaffold in combination with other regenerative therapies, hyaluronic acid can support cell growth and tissue regeneration.

- *Gene therapy:* Experimental approaches using gene editing tools to modify gene expression in the endometrial lining are being explored to enhance regenerative capabilities, though this field is still in its infancy.

CHALLENGES AND FUTURE DIRECTIONS

Despite the promising potential of these therapies, several challenges remain. Variability in treatment protocols, lack of standardized dosages, and limited large-scale clinical trials hinder widespread adoption. Future research should focus on:

- Establishing standardized treatment protocols.
- Conducting large, randomized controlled trials to validate efficacy.
- Exploring combinatory approaches to enhance therapeutic outcomes.

CONCLUSION

Regenerative therapies such as PRP, stem cells, and exosomes represent a frontier in treating thin endometrium, offering new hope for patients with challenging reproductive conditions. While further research is essential, these innovative approaches have the potential to significantly improve endometrial receptivity and fertility outcomes, marking a new era in reproductive medicine.

REFERENCES

1. Abrao MS, et al. The impact of platelet-rich plasma on thin endometrium: A meta-analysis. Reprod Med. 2023;47(3):258-65.
2. Zhao X, et al. Menstrual blood-derived stem cells in the treatment of Asherman's syndrome: A clinical trial. Fertil Steril. 2022;118(5):1020-8.
3. Chen Y, et al. Exosomes as a regenerative therapy for thin endometrium: A systematic review. Gynecol Res. 2023;56(1):74-81.